*Handbook of*

# *Neurological Examination*

*and*

# *Case Recording*

D. Denny-Brown, M.D., was Putnam Professor of Neurology,
Emeritus, Harvard Medical School

D. M. Dawson, M.D., is Associate Professor of Neurology,
Harvard Medical School

H. R. Tyler, M.D., is Professor of Neurology,
Harvard Medical School

# Handbook of

# Neurological Examination

## and

## Case Recording

Third Edition

**D. Denny-Brown, M.D.**

**D. M. Dawson, M.D.**

**H. R. Tyler, M.D.**

HARVARD UNIVERSITY PRESS

CAMBRIDGE, MASSACHUSETTS

and LONDON, ENGLAND

1982

**Library of Congress Cataloging in Publication Data**

Denny-Brown, D. (Derek), 1901-
  Handbook of neurological examination and case recording.
    1. Neurologic examination—Handbooks, manuals, etc.    2. Neu-
rologic examination—Case studies—Handbooks, manuals, etc.
I. Dawson, D. M.    II. Tyler, H. R.    III. Title.    [DNLM:
1. Medical history taking.    2. Neurologic examination.    3. Nervous
system diseases—Diagnosis.    WL 141 D412h]
RC348.D45   1982              616.8'0475              81-13315
ISBN 0-674-37101-1                                    AACR2

### Note on the Third Edition

This book should provide the initiate with the basic material for evaluating a patient with a disorder affecting the nervous system. The separation between history and physical examination is artificial. The astute clinician notes the significance of the symptoms he is eliciting and their anatomical and physiological importance. He knows what information he must seek from his examination before doing it, and he proceeds in a fashion to elicit it. Similarly, unexpected findings in examination frequently require more questioning or modifying one's "set." How one goes about this can influence whether or not the patient will follow the physician's advice. The neurological examination is eminently suited to answer the question "Where is the lesion?" Taken in context with the history, it then becomes more logical to ask "what" is wrong with the patient.

In preparing a new edition, we have revised some sections in which our viewpoint has changed in the last ten years. The "art" of the examination does not change, but the background information and procedures continually evolve. Minor changes and corrections have been made. We feel strongly that the need of both junior and senior students is for a manual, small enough to fit into the pocket of a ward jacket, dealing with the basic facts of clinical examination and initial approaches to patient problems.

## Foreword to the First Published Edition

This handbook is written for senior students and house officers to introduce them to standard neurological methods. There are many ways of eliciting the facts of clinical neurology and of recording them, and each clinician in time works out a method based on those ways and means which he has found to serve him well. But at first it is essential to select a methodical procedure, for the multiplicity of signs is as confusing as their different values in interpretation. It is hoped that the following pages will serve both to present reliable methods and their usage in clinical neurology and to stimulate a greater uniformity in presentation of the facts on case records.

The booklet was first issued in March 1942 in a private printing for the Neurological Unit. It has been completely revised, and in part, particularly the sections dealing with lumbar and cistern puncture, rewritten. I am greatly indebted to Drs. Raymond D. Adams and Harry L. Kozol for their advice and assistance.

D. Denny-Brown

April 1946
Neurological Unit, Boston City Hospital
Department of Neurology, Harvard Medical School

# Contents

## *Introduction*

## *Methods of Examination and Recording*

*Special Investigations*

*Tables and Figures*

## Introduction

### The History

In neurology a great deal depends on an accurate history. Each symptom has potential physiological or anatomical value. The process of collecting symptoms is not passive but is one of interpreting and clarifying. Further information enhances or contributes to the meaning or validity of symptoms and must be sought by inquiry. A good physician uses his own background and experience in eliciting the maximal potential information from the patient and his family.

In any patient with a disorder of the central nervous system, which may have associated mental changes, it is critical to seek an independent history and confirmation of the factual details. The sources of the history and the examiner's overall estimate of their value should be noted early in the written record.

In the history, ascertaining the timing and speed of events is of great value in diagnosis. Of pain, one should inquire systematically and record its nature (dull, aching, sharp, shooting, burning, tingling, etc.), its distribution, its duration (continuous, paroxysmal, repetitive, etc.), its frequency, its relation to time of day, to posture, and to other factors, such as movement or coughing, and to other symptoms. The same data on nature, distribution, and relativity can be systematically elicited of an abnormal movement, a vertigo, or a clouding of consciousness. The patient's statement of attacks of loss of consciousness, fits, etc., of defect in memory, or of mental abnormality are recorded for what they are worth. Only with experience can the physician assess the value of the patient's description of such states. He will cross-question the patient as to the circumstances, attempting to decide whether the patient's behavior and the mode of onset and recovery from the episode were consistent with his supposed condition. He then asks what other people told the patient about his behavior and seeks to get a history from some witness of the event. With experience, the physician will learn some differences between the amnesias of hysteria and of coma.

A regular order in recording both the history and the results of examination is of value both in ensuring completeness and in facilitating subsequent reference. The following order is suggested.

1. The patient's complaint, a brief statement of the problem, preferably in the patient's own words.

2. Present illness in chronological order, ideally in the patient's own words. Few patients, however, keep sufficiently to the point, and many questions are necessary. A compromise is therefore followed; the history is written objectively in the third person, and answers to the examiner's questions are woven into the description. If, however, the examiner asks leading questions about some important point (questions the examiner feels would suggest ideas to a suggestible person), the description should quote the patient's own words. The examiner then checks this statement by ask-

ing, if "dizziness" is mentioned, for example, whether the patient or things around him seemed to be spinning and in which direction, and will then endeavor to reach a conclusion as to whether the patient was suffering from true vertigo or simply from a sensation of uncertainty or from faintness.

Special inquiry should always be made about the following symptoms which are important in a neurological case study:

Sudden disturbances in consciousness
Convulsions
Headache
Loss of vision
Diplopia
Deafness and tinnitus
Vertigo
Nausea and vomiting
Dysphagia
Speech disorder, either in the understanding and use of words, or articulation
Weakness, stiffness, or paralysis of the limbs
Pains and paresthesias
Disturbances in control of rectal and vesical sphincters.

The nature and degree of the patient's anxieties should be ascertained, and the relationship, if any, between dramatic events in his medical history and emotional stress in his daily life.

Patients often describe in great detail the numerous doctors they have seen, the hospitals they have attended, and what was said or done to them, without mentioning what was happening to their pain or other complaint in this period. Only repeated questions (which need not be mentioned in the record) will elicit this more essential information.

Any information from earlier examination or medical

records should be abstracted and added at the end of the recorded history of the present illness.

3. Family history—any known history of mental or nervous breakdown, suicide, headaches, fits or faints, or paralysis should be especially solicited. Significant medical disorders in the family should always be noted (diabetes, hypertension, cancer, etc.).

4. Marital history.

5. Social history.

6. Occupational history, including level of education.

7. Past medical history and system review.

### The Record of Neurological Examination

In medicine, as in any other branch of science, next to the ability to observe matters of fact, the ability to keep adequate record of such observations is very important. Of each observation the student must learn what is significant and then how to communicate his observation in clear yet simple terms to others. Description should be in positive terms; to say that the pulse is "somewhat irregular" is obviously inadequate. A patient is not necessarily either emaciated or obese, excited or depressed. Learn to describe intermediate variations. On the other hand, an adequate description does not need to cover every possible variable. Only constant practice brings facility in description, conciseness with relevant detail. Avoid phrases such as "tends to" or "is suggestive of." An ounce of fact is worth ten of noncommittal statement.

The purpose of the record is to give a concise description of the patient's condition as it appears to the observer. An attempt should be made to convey an impression of the patient, for instance, whether he is quiet and reserved or talkative and agitated, whether introspective and overanxious because of his illness or euphoric and unconcerned, intelligent or not, cooperative in examination or resentful. This should come at the beginning of the description. The order of description is important in that uniformity greatly facilitates subsequent analysis of case histories. The following order is therefore suggested.

1. General impression of the patient's awareness of his surroundings, his ability to cooperate in examination, and his ability to converse. Mention here his personality, mannerisms, any obvious abnormal movements or attitude, or abnormality in gait.

2. Mental status. The use of simple tests for memory and intelligence (digit retention, serial 7 subtraction, events in the day's newspaper, names of presidents or cities) is recommended in all cerebral affections, for they give a good general guide to day-to-day, or month-to-month, changes in the patient's condition. If there is any intellectual defect, a full mental status should be attempted and recorded here.

3. Enumeration of abnormalities in the cranial nerves in order from olfactory to hypoglossal nerve.

4. Motor function. Upper limbs, neck and trunk, and lower limbs, in that order, describing abnormalities of posture, power of movement, development and bulk of the muscles, coordination, and resistance to passive movement (postural tone) in each part.

5. The essential reflexes, tabulated with responses on right and left sides indicated, and any other unusual reflex movement that is observed, concluding with a remark on the state of the sphincters.

6. Sensation. Refer to a chart but also give a brief description. Tabulate the findings under touch, pain, temperature, position sense, vibration, two-point discrimination, tactile localization, and stereognosis.

7. The results of palpation and other search for tender-

ness of neuromuscular and ligamentous structures, and of special tests for meningitis, sciatic tenderness, etc., also any pertinent observations (palpation-auscultation) concerning the vascular system, including specific arteries to the face and head and blood pressure in the two arms.

8. Description of general examination, including cardio-vascular, respiratory, alimentary, renal, and endocrine systems.

9. Record of special investigations, such as lumbar puncture, X-rays, electroencephalography, record of muscular excitability, biopsy, etc.

10. A brief general impression as a result of your history and examination, stating the nature of the disability, your deduction as to the probable location and nature of the lesion, and lastly, your plan of investigation and therapy.

## Progress Notes

As the case investigation progresses or as the history or findings are modified, there should be a description in the form of progress notes. This serves the purposes of communicating to other members of the clinical team, recording information as a logical record of data, and enlarging the data base. It also serves as a medical-legal record, and any writing should be done with the knowledge that such records will be available to the patient and legal representative as well as to medical personnel.

## Methods of Examination and Recording

Awareness, Personality, and
General Defects, Including Gait

*Awareness.* Too often the clinical record omits to state the important fact that the patient is semicomatose, or in coma. General awareness should be stated at the very beginning. Some difficulty attaches to the definition of "unconsciousness," and it is best, as with many other clinical terms, to describe what happens and not use a term that is part observation, part deduction and has no absolute definition.

States of impairment of consciousness are judged by the reaction of the patient to his environment. Insensibility is deep when the patient no longer makes any reaction to painful stimulus. If painful stimulus elicits only a primitive movement (corneal reflex, withdrawal of a limb or part of a limb), and no other stimulus elicits any response, the condition is described as coma (see section on examination of the patient in coma). A full definition is "the absence of any psychologically understandable response to external stimuli or inner need."*

*See Fred Plum and Jerome Posner, *Diagnosis of Stupor and Coma*, 3rd ed. (Philadelphia: F. A. Davis, 1980).

If some psychologically understandable response (e.g., change of expression, attempt to brush away an offending object, or restlessness due to distended bladder) is present, but elicited only by painful or disagreeable stimuli such as pinching the skin or shaking the patient vigorously, the condition is called semicoma.

Lesser degrees of clouding of consciousness are termed confusion, which covers "impaired capacity to think clearly and with customary rapidity and to perceive, respond to and remember current stimuli." This includes disorientation. When confusion is associated with reduction in spontaneous activity, the state may be called apathy or stupor, depending on its degree. The following degrees of confusion may be defined:

*Severe.* The patient is in general inaccessible but occasionally responds adequately to simple commands, forcibly given and if necessary reinforced by adequate gestures, e.g., "Put out your tongue," "Shut your eyes."

*Moderate.* The patient, though out of touch with his surroundings, can give relevant answers to simple questions such as "What work do you do?" "How old are you?" "Where do you live?"

*Mild.* There is a defect in alertness, comprehension, and/or judgment, but the patient retains the capacity for coherent conversation and appropriate behavior.

Confusion which has been gradually lessening in degree usually ceases the moment the patient recovers full orientation in time.

The patient with disturbance of alertness requires special types of examinations, as he cannot be expected to cooperate.

*Personality.* Some attempt should be made to convey the personality of the patient in the record, as has been mentioned. This should include his reaction to, and attitude about, his illness and disability.

*General defects.* This means the first general impression of the disability, if it is obvious as you view the patient for the first time. Thus, if the patient's left arm lies limply by his side, or if he is convulsed by some recurring spasm, or if he stops speaking and grimaces from pain, the mention of it at this point gives a general view of the abnormality before your detailed examination proceeds to define its nature. If the patient appears healthy and without any disorder, this should also be stated. He may appear to be in excellent health until he begins to stand up or walk, so a brief statement as to station, gait, and speech should be made here, for the same purpose of defining the general facts of observation before proceeding to the particular.

*Gait.* If the patient cannot stand, attempt to decide whether it is because of weakness or of unsteadiness. *If he can stand* but is unsteady, note if he tends to fall consistently in one direction and if the unsteadiness is increased when his eyes are closed (Romberg's test). *If he can walk,* does he deviate or reel, does he swing his limbs naturally? He may move his legs too loosely, sometimes lifting them too high, sometimes stamping, usually on a wide base (as occurs in both sensory and cerebellar ataxia). If there is a foot-drop, the foot is lifted unusually high to allow the toes to clear the ground. If there is weakness in flexion of the hip, the forward movement of the step is slow. If in addition there is stiffness of the leg and weakness in flexion of the knee (as in spastic weakness), the pelvis is tilted at each step and the leg circumducted to clear the ground. In that case, the toe of the shoe will be worn down.

If the patient walks with some exaggerated slowness and

staggering toward support, he may have lost confidence in his legs. Long hesitation before advancing each foot and then a sudden shuffling movement, associated with elaborate balancing movements of the trunk and upper limbs, is characteristic of a pure loss of confidence (hysterical gait).

Lack of swinging of the arms when walking may be due to rigidity or spasticity, but in the absence of these abnormalities it is seen in cerebellar disease on the same side. Loss of equilibrium when turning may be due to ataxia, vertigo, or rigidity. Advanced Parkinsonism may result in rapid small steps because of difficulty in controlling the center of gravity, owing to rigidity.

Only with experience can the lesser degrees of these variations of gait be recognized, and the importance of their recognition as physical signs of nervous disease cannot be overestimated.

To give greater prominence to defects that are very slight, have the patient walk with eyes open and shut, walk a line heel-to-toe (tandem gait), or walk on the heels or toes, with sudden turning, starting, and stopping.

The following are characteristic disorders of gait:

1. Hemiplegic gait—circumduction of leg, stiff knee, scraping.
2. Spastic paraplegic gait—slow, stiff, with tilting pelvis and delayed flexion of hip.
3. Steppage gait—flopping feet, lifted too high.
4. Sensory ataxia—wide base, uneven steps, stamping.
5. Cerebellar—wide base, irregularity, deviation or reeling, staggering on turning.
6. Parkinsonism (festinating)—stooped posture, short steps, acceleration, chasing center of gravity.

7. Hysterical gaits—inconsistent with other ability to move the limbs, exaggerated balancing.

## Intellectual Function

Diseases of the brain are often manifested by disorders of orientation, memory, and judgment, and these are as much clinical factual findings as are the changes in physical signs. In more complicated states, change in mood and personality has also to be assessed. For general neurological examination a short form of mental status should be used.

The examination of a patient's mental status requires a combination of sympathetic interest and critical detachment. On the one hand it is important to encourage the patient to talk freely and honestly. On the other hand it is important to assay his statements carefully. The relationship between physician and patient is a subtle one, friendly but not familiar, and exemplifies the art of interpersonal relationships. In trying to gain information concerning specific subjects, the physician should be relatively direct, yet not blunt or abrupt. Judicious direction of an informal conversation can cover all the data required for a dependable approximation of the mental status.

Specific observations are useful in attempting to quantify and characterize defects. The following aspects of mental status are worth documenting and making specific observations that can be recorded.

*Sensorium and Intellectual Status*

*Attention.* To what extent does the patient show and main-

tain attention to your examination? If necessary, test attention and ability to concentrate by reading a story to the
patient and noting whether he remembers it. Another simple
but effective test is to read a series of digits or letters to the
patient and have him raise his finger every time a particular
one (say 7 or R) is spoken.

Many patients who are hospitalized with medical or surgi-
cal illnesses, in pain, or sedated with drugs are inattentive,
which markedly alters their capacity to perform on tests.
Patients who are severely inattentive are also—probably as a
result—disoriented to time.

*Orientation.* Record the patient's answers to questions
about his name and identity, the place where he is, the time of
day, and the date. Does he think there is anything unusual in
the way that time seems to pass?

*Memory.* Remote memory may be tested by comparing the
patient's account of his life with that given by others or by
examining his account for gaps or inconsistencies. Information which he gives about his earlier life, personality, school
and work experiences, etc., should not be inserted here but
included as a supplementary part of the history, with its
source indicated.

Do you have a good memory?

Where and when were you born?

How old does that make you?

Where and how long did you go to school?

What year did you graduate? At what age?

What jobs have you had? When?

When were you married? At what age?

What are the names, ages, and years of birth of your
   children?

What are your parents' names? If they are dead, when
   did they die? At what age?

To test intermediate memory, ask the patient to give a chronological account of his illness, with dates. Can he give the events of the last five years in his own life, as well as general events?

There should be special inquiry about recent events, such as his admission to hospital and happenings in the ward since.

What time did you come to the hospital?

How did you come here?

With whom?

What did you have at your last meal? (Be sure the examiner knows.)

Note whether there is selective impairment of memory for special incidents, periods, recent or remote happenings, or whether the impairment is generalized and extends through both recent and remote events, consistent or scattered. Does the patient confabulate? ("What did you do yesterday?" "Didn't I see you in the street?")

A patient who is inattentive will have difficulty with memory testing because the questions do not sink in; recent memory is particularly affected.

*Retention and immediate recall.* Digit retention is a useful test. "To see how your memory is," (or, "To test your concentration which you complained about,") "I am going to say some numbers. After I am through, I would like you to repeat them just as I did." Name the digits one per second, beginning with 3 or 4, and proceed as far as the patient can go. Record the exact responses, which are important for transpositions, etc.

Another test is to give the patient a complicated sentence and ask him to repeat it, or give him a simple address, such as 35 North Broadway, Philadelphia, and the names of two objects, such as pencil and table, and a color, and tell him he will be asked to repeat these in three minutes. Test after three minutes have elapsed. Also ask the patient to repeat the doctor's name after some minutes.

Read aloud a brief story, then have the patient repeat it and give its meaning.

*Calculations.* 1. The 100 – 7 test: Ask the patient to subtract 7 from 100 and to continue subtracting 7 from the result. The observer should make certain that the test is understood and may use any form of encouragement short of giving the patient the actual number. The patient's responses are recorded, along with the time taken to complete the test (average time is 40-50 seconds).

2. "Count from 1 to 20 and backward from 20 down to 1." Record the time.

3. "What would be the interest on $200 at 10% for 18 months?"

4. "How much is 3 times 16?" (and other simple multiplications).

*Grasp of general information.* The following questions relating to general information may be used:

The name of the president and his immediate predecessors

The name of the mayor of the patient's city or the governor of the state

The capitals of France, West Germany, Italy, and the United States

The five largest cities in America

The dates of Washington's Birthday, Christmas

Dates of beginning and end of World Wars I and II

The names of three large rivers

What are the colors of traffic lights? What are they for?

*Special tests.* In addition to the above, the patient may be given numerous additional tests, such as word definitions, interpretations of fables and proverbs, detection of absurdities, abstraction of likenesses, etc. Such tests are particularly useful to demonstrate the presence of slight but definite defects in judgment and intellectual acuity, such as may be found in the early stages of dementia or as a residue of severe head injury or anoxic encephalopathy. The tests are not intended to estimate general intelligence but to see whether there has been any falling away from the patient's former presumptive level of knowledge and capacity.

*Insight and judgment.* What is the patient's attitude to his present state? Does he regard it as an illness and needing treatment? Is he aware of his mistakes made spontaneously or in response to tests? How does he regard them and other details of his condition? Does he recognize and acknowledge any special incapacity he may have? Does he exaggerate or minimize its importance? What is his attitude to recovery? How does he regard previous experiences, psychological symptoms, etc., that are relevant? What is his attitude toward social, financial, domestic, ethical problems? Is his judgment good? What does he propose to do when he has left the hospital?

The tests described above will give a general picture of the patient's cognitive and intellectual function. The results must be considered in the perspective of the patient's illness and medical care and are not a formal ritual to be gone through for the sake of completing a record. They are designed to show the examiner whether the patient's intellectual functions have been affected, as compared with his previous level of function.

If you believe that the patient has specific language or behavioral defects related to focal cerebral cortical lesion, see the descriptions of further testing in the sections on aphasia, perceptive disorder, agnosia, and apraxia.

## Cranial Nerve Function

*Olfactory nerve.* Sense of smell should be tested by obliterating one nostril and holding the mouth of a small bottle containing cotton soaked with oil of lemon, cloves, camphor, or coffee, under the other nostril. At the bedside, soap and toothpaste are usually available and satisfactory. If the patient is unable to distinguish odors in one or both sides, note if the airway is clear. Record results by stating which odors are named correctly and which incorrectly, in each nostril. Note that ammonia vapor or other pungent substances are not a test of olfactory function.

*Vision.* State visual acuity using the standard chart for 20 meters, as follows:

$$V.O.D. = \frac{20}{size\ read}$$

$$V.O.S. = \frac{20}{size\ read}$$

Indicate whether improvement is obtained by correction. If distant vision is good, but ability to read is impaired, also record result of test with Jaeger test type, stating smallest type read by patient at usual reading distance or with reading glasses if necessary.

The results of any test of the visual fields should next be recorded and the method stated. Thus, "Confrontation test showed inability to appreciate finger movement in the upper quadrant of the left field on each side. On the perimeter the patient was found to have a complete left homonymous hemianopia to 1° object (see attached perimeter charts)."

The confrontation test is important in testing all forms of cerebral disease and should be an integral part of the neurological examination. Performed carelessly, it is of little value, but if done carefully it can pick up even small defects which are difficult to show by other means. Sit facing the patient and direct him to look at one of your eyes (right eye if you are testing his left, and vice versa). Have him cover, but not press on, the eye not being tested. Hold up both hands and have him point to the side on which he sees a finger move. Test his ability to see small movements in each quadrant of each field. Try movement on both sides at once, for parietal lobe or large diffuse lesions sometimes cause failure to appreciate movement in the field if presented concurrently with movement on the opposite side (attention hemianopia), whereas movement on the affected side alone is appreciated correctly. Then proceed to test for detailed outline of the defect by means of a white test object on a rod. The coarsest test for vision is sense of movement in the field of vision (the last to be affected, the first to recover).

If any defect is found in the confrontation test, the fields must be charted on a perimeter. Every case of suspected cerebral disease should have the fields charted, whether a defect is suspected or not. For charting fields on the 330 mm. perimeter the white objects subtending 1° and ½° are standard, and they must be moved slowly. The smaller the object, the more sensitive the test. With some gross defects in vision, only 1° is reliable. Always state the size of object used on the perimeter chart, either in degrees or as size in mm. over distance in mm. (e.g. 5/2000).

If the defect encroaches on the center of the visual field or affects only the center of the field (central or paracentral scotoma) it may be charted on a one-meter tangent screen with great accuracy.* It is as well to gain a rough idea of the dimensions of the defect by confrontation test with a small white object first. In charting a scotoma, begin in the center of the defect and move outward until the object is seen. If the loss of vision is such that the patient is unable to fix on a small white object, use two strips of paper or tape, crossing at right angles in the center of the screen, and tell him to look at the point where he judges them to cross, or on the perimeter get him to put his finger on the fixation point and look where the tip of his finger is. In all perimetry the patient's eye must be watched *all the time* the object is being moved to make sure his eye does not deviate.

The state of the optic fundi should next be noted. State whether the disc edges are sharply defined, and if not, whether there is any swelling. The degree of swelling may be measured by adding plus lenses until the retina is out of focus, then lessening the value until the first part of the disc is in focus. Then do the same for some small vessel near the macula. The difference in lens value gives the swelling in diopters. Reliable measurements require practice in relaxing accommodation. Note the color of the disc, and if pale, whether you can see the natural rim of pinkness all around the central pit, and if the natural markings of the physiological cup are obliterated. Note the size and regularity of the retinal vessels, whether the arteries nip the veins where they cross, and if there are any hemorrhages or white exudate to be seen. Beware of reporting myelinated nerve fibers as exudate or swelling. If there is vascular hypertension, note especially if the retinal arteries show narrowed segments. If so, make a

*For full description of screen perimetry see D. O. Harrington, *The Visual Fields,* 3rd ed. (St. Louis: C. V. Mosby, 1971).

diagram showing the two main arteries, upper and lower, and the nasal and temporal branch of each, with the location of the narrowed segment indicated. If there is a question of diabetes, look especially for the little dark red rounded aneurysmal dilatations. If there is a question of cerebral vascular malformation, look for abnormally tortuous or beaded retinal vessels and any abnormality at the termination of these. Note any abnormal pigmentation and its distribution.

Note any opacities in the ocular media.

*Third, fourth, and sixth cranial serves.* It is convenient to group all these nerves together. First describe the pupils— their size, any irregularity or inequality in shape—then their reaction to light. If one fails to react briskly to light, does it react to light in the other eye (consensual reaction)? Then describe the reaction to convergence. Be careful that the amount of light is the same as before convergence.

Next describe any retraction, lag, or drooping of the lids, and note any corresponding staring expression with retraction, or compensatory overaction of frontalis muscle with ptosis. Do not mistake asymmetrical folding of the upper lid for ptosis. One or both upper lids may be retracted, revealing the whole iris.

Then describe any lack of parallelism between the visual axes at rest and in following the examiner's finger. If there is a defect in any movement, state the direction in which movement is defective, in each eye. This may be so slight that no defect in movement of the eyes is seen by the observer despite the patient's complaint of diplopia. In that case state in which direction of movement of the eyes the separation of images occurs, remembering that it is the false image that is overprojected in the direction of movement. If necessary, place a red glass in front of one eye to identify the eye responsible for each image.

Any regular rhythmical movement of the eyes (nystagmus) should be described. Does it consistently have a fast component in one direction and slower return in the other (jerk nystagmus), or is it oscillating, with the same speed in each direction (pendular nystagmus)? Such movements are a fault in fixation, oscillating if related to retinal causes, and caused by drift in the direction of the slow component if due to brain stem disease. The rapid component is the compensating movement. The direction of such nystagmus is that of the rapid component, for this is the direction of movement that is faulty. Thus, if the patient is requested to look at an object farther to the right than the eyes can normally deviate, his eyes move slowly away from extreme deviation, returning in a series of rapid jerks. This is a normal phenomenon and has no neurologic significance. When the eyes fail in this way to maintain deviation within the normal range of movement, the nystagmus becomes a significant neurologic sign. Damage to the brain stem causes nystagmus that is slower and coarser to the side of the lesion. Vertical nystagmus is typically caused by brain stem disease. Irritation of the labyrinth causes a deviation of the eyes to the opposite side, and the associated nystagmus has a rotary component.

The smoothness of ocular following should be noted, because a breakdown of pursuit movements into saccadic jerks may indicate brain stem or cerebellar disorder.

Congenital nystagmus is usually an irregular oscillating movement related to rapid fatigue of macular fixation (defect in retinal pigment).

The range of eye motion in response to command, following, and head turning (so-called doll's head) should be noted, and movements to each direction compared.

Undue prominence of one or both eyes (proptosis, exophthalmos) should be noted here. Some estimate of the degree can be obtained by looking down on the patient's face from above, noting how prominent the cornea is on each side in relation to the eyebrow as the patient looks upward. Beware of being misled by undue thickness or redundant folds in the eyelids.

Note to what extent the patient can converge the two eyes on an approaching finger.

*Fifth nerve.* Feel the two masseter muscles when the patient bites hard and note if they contract equally or are wasted, and note if the mandible deviates to one side (weak pterygoid muscles) when he attempts to lower the jaw against your resistance.

Describe here any loss of sensation to touch or pin prick on the face, testing all three divisions of the fifth nerve separately.

Note the state of the corneal reflex, elicited by touching the cornea slowly with a wisp of cotton while the patient's gaze is directed upward. It is important to be sure the stimulus is on the cornea, not the sclera.

*Seventh nerve.* Note any asymmetry of the face at rest and in willed movement, such as showing the teeth, shutting the eyes, frowning, smiling, and in emotional and associated movements such as occur with spontaneous smiling, speech, and wincing from a pin prick. If weakness is present, is it more obvious in the lower facial muscles than in closure of the eyes? Slight degrees of generalized weakness may be emphasized by an attempt to frown or raise the eyebrows.

Is there any spasm of the facial muscles or tremor? Slight tremors can be seen more easily in the eyelids when the patient closes them lightly. Perioral tremor may appear only in the course of movements of the lips, and be absent with full movement.

If there is interference with cortical control of facial movement, reflex pouting or sucking occurs when the lip is stroked. A tap on a finger that stretches the facial muscles then usually elicits a facial jerk.

Sense of taste on the anterior two thirds of the tongue may be lost from affection of the seventh nerve proximal to the chorda tympani branch. It is tested by dabbing a very small amount of sugar, salt, or vinegar with a moist applicator on the coarser folds on the lateral edge of the tongue about halfway back from the tip. The patient should be instructed to put his tongue out to the opposite side and to nod if he tastes anything, then say what the taste is. There is little taste near the tip of the tongue.

*Eighth nerve.* Give some measure of hearing, such as "hears whispered voice at three feet in each ear," or "hears watch at two feet in right ear and six inches in left." Is air conduction greater than bone conduction? (Rinne test). Is the sound of a tuning fork applied to the center of the forehead referred to one side? (Weber test). Hearing should be tested with high, middle, and low frequency tones. A tuning fork usually will test only lower tones, which are affected late in the course of most neurological diseases. Speech and watch tick can be easily added to the observations. State here if the tympanic membrane is of normal appearance.

No labyrinthine test is necessary in routine examination, although it may be desirable in evaluating a comatose patient, to see the intactness of the vestibular oculomotor connections.

*Ninth and tenth nerves.* Movements of the palate during articulation will show the pulling of the uvula to the stronger side. Does touching the mucous membrane of the pharynx evoke a contraction (gag reflex)? If the voice is brassy or hoarse, inspect the vocal cords.

*Eleventh nerve.* Contraction of the sternomastoid muscle on turning the head to each side against resistance and of the trapezius in shrugging the shoulders against resistance should be estimated, and any wasting or spasm noted.

*Twelfth nerve.* The patient is asked to protrude the tongue fully, and any deviation from the midline and any atrophy is noted. Deviation of the mandible due to affection of the fifth nerve or of the lips due to weakness of the facial musculature must be discounted. If there is doubt as to weakness in tongue movement, get the patient to push the tongue against each cheek in turn. If the protruded tongue is tremulous, is the tremor rhythmical? Small irregular twitchings or jerks of the muscles are not unusual in normal people. The little agitated flickerings (fibrillation) of true atrophy are best seen as the tongue lies in the floor of the mouth. They are usually best seen on the lateral aspects in areas of slight atrophy.

Considerable difficulty in articulation of lingual and labial sounds may be due to bilateral weakness which is only slight in degree. Fibrillation and atrophy are then of the greatest significance as confirmatory signs of lower motor neuron lesion. Stiffness of the labiolingual muscles, either from bilateral damage to corticobulbar tracts (pseudobulbar paralysis) or from the rigidity of Parkinsonism, will also cause a slurring of speech with little objective change in the movements of the tongue. This can be confirmed by evidence of spasticity or rigidity in other muscles.

The peculiar feature of cerebellar dysarthria is a fairly rhythmical grouping of syllables. It is heard as "scanning" in disturbance of cerebellar connections in the brain stem, as in multiple sclerosis, or in a slower halting, often with explosive utterance of syllables, in cerebellar disease.

## Motor Function

The description should begin with the upper limbs, then proceed to the neck and trunk, and then to the lower limbs.

The motor exam should begin by first noting any abnormality of posture and any tremor or spasm observed while the limb is at rest. This is an excellent rapid screening test. Then proceed to record any abnormality, change in posture, or drifting while the patient's arms are outstretched in front. This gives an initial general idea of the extent of weakness, wasting, tremor, etc. In the legs the same purpose is served by asking the patient to raise first one and then the other whole leg from the bed or couch.

*Movement.* The power of movement is tested independently for each movement at each joint or for each muscle, depending on what one is looking for (see Table 1). This can be rapidly performed if done in a routine order. If weakness is patchy, it is well to tabulate the joints and possible movements as illustrated:

|  |  | *Right* | *Left* |
|---|---|---|---|
| *Wrist:* | dorsiflexion | 5 (100%) | 0 |
|  | palmarflexion | 4 | 1 |
|  | adduction (radial flexion) | 3 | 2 |
|  | abduction (ulnar flexion) | 1 | 0 |

On a 5-point scale, 0 = no contraction, 1 = a very feeble

flicker of contraction, 2 = a weak contraction not sufficient to overcome gravity, 3 = a weak contraction that can counteract gravity but is easily overcome, 4 = fair but not full strength, and 5 = full power of contraction. Since some schemes use 4 for complete paralysis, it is better to write 100% as well as 5 at least once in your table.

The earliest upper motor neuron weakness is found in the dorsiflexors of wrist and ankle.

The contraction of the abdominal muscles may be estimated by watching them as the patient coughs or raises his head from the pillow. The intercostals are felt by the fingertips during inspiration and cough, and diaphragmatic movements shown by percussion or, better, fluoroscopy. Movements of the spinal muscles are best observed by making the patient bend forward, then backward when stripped. If the history suggests a nerve or a root lesion, one can perform the muscle examination in the fashion that is most logical to the history, examining those muscles which will give the appropriate anatomical information.

In some affections (e.g., Parkinsonism) the power of resisting passive movement is strong, while the speed and extent of movement is lessened by rigidity of the muscles. In suggested weakness (hysteria), the patient performs a movement feebly and unsteadily but can offer resistance proportionate to the full force of countermovement made by the examiner (i.e., loss of movement but not loss of contraction.) Collapsing weakness, in which the patient "gives way," is also characteristic of functional weakness or pain preventing full cooperation.

The ability to relax a contraction promptly is seldom affected. It is delayed a little in myxedema. It is greatly impaired in myotonia, where any very strong contraction (grasp,

Table 1. Segmental innervation of muscles.

| Region | Muscle | Nerve |
|---|---|---|
| Neck | Trapezius | C2, 3,* 4 |
| | Sternomastoid | C1, 2 |
| | Diaphragm | C3, 4, 5 |
| Shoulder | Supra- and infra-spinatus | C5,* 6 |
| | Deltoid | C5, 6 |
| | Serratus magnus | C5, 6, 7 |
| Arm | Biceps, brachialis, and brachioradialis | C5, 6 |
| | Triceps | C6, 7* |
| Forearm | Extensors of wrist | C6,* 7, 8 |
| | Extensors of metacarpophalangeal joints | C6, 7,* 8 |
| | Flexors of wrist | C7, 8,* D1 |
| | Radial deviation of wrist | C6, 7* |
| | Ulnar deviation of wrist | C7, 8,* D1 |
| | Supination | C5,* 6 |
| | Pronation | C6, 7,* 8 |
| Hand | Lumbricals, interossei, opposition of thumb | C8, D1* |
| | Abductor and flexor pollicis brevis | C7, 8* |
| Pelvic Girdle | Iliopsoas | D12, L1,* 2,* 3 |
| | Glutei | L4, 5,* S1 |
| Thigh | Quadriceps | L2, 3,* 4 |
| | Adductors | L2, 3, 4 |
| | Semi-tend. and Semi-memb. | L4, 5, S1 |
| | Biceps femoris | L5,* S1, 2 |
| Leg | Gastrocnemius and soleus | L5, S1,* 2 |
| | Tibialis anterior | L4, 5 |
| | Peronei | L5, S1 |
| Foot | Short plantar muscles | S1, 2 |
| Perineal muscles | | S3, 4, 5 |
| Bladder | Smooth muscle | S2, 3 |

*Innervation is chiefly from one motor root.

or closure of the eyes) is followed by a long delay in relaxation. This delay is lessened by repeated contraction of the same muscles. Percussion of the muscle (most prominently the thenar eminence and the tongue) then should elicit a similarly prolonged contraction. Delay in relaxation of the grasp may also be caused by lesion of the opposite frontal lobe, but is then associated with the positive grasping reaction to a distally moving stimulus in the palm of the hand (grasp reflex) that is responsible for the continued response to grasp.

*Atrophy.* Note the bulk of the muscles and the relationship of smallness (atrophy) to loss of power of contraction. List the muscle groups that show atrophy and weakness, for the distribution of these is significant. In general emaciation or disuse atrophy, the muscle still contracts strongly. In recent lower motor neuron weakness the power of contraction is small in relation to the size of the muscle, whereas in longstanding lower motor neuron affections the power of contraction of the residual muscle is surprisingly good.

Watch for small, flickering, involuntary contraction of groups of muscle fibers (fasciculation). In atrophic muscles, residual normal motor units are commonly coarse and when activated show a tremulous twitching of the part of the muscle in which they lie. This type of twitching (contraction fasciculation) is abolished by complete relaxation and renewed in the same place in the muscle belly with each contraction. More important is the irregular repetition of single twitches in one or other part of the muscle, with many seconds or minutes elapsing before another twitch recurs in exactly the same place in the muscle. This is true fasciculation and is due to an abnormal impulse from a diseased anterior horn cell in motor neuron disease. Repetitive fasciculations in the same spot which occur in bursts often are seen in root lesions. To be fully significant, true fasciculation should be associated with atrophy and weakness. Another type of twitching, benign fasciculation, is commonly confused with true fasciculation. This is repetitive in the same fasciculus, is usually coarser, and is not associated with weakness or atrophy. It is a small muscle cramp. Irregular undulation of the surface of muscles (myokymia) is a mild form of tetany, where each abnormal contraction is slower than true fasciculation.

The excitability of muscles may be diminished or increased. A rough test for this is the response to a tap on the muscle substance with a percussion hammer. Normal muscles show a local twitch in the fasciculi under the point struck. In emaciated persons some continued flickering may occur for a few seconds but is of no value as a diagnostic sign. Atrophic muscle gives a feeble contraction, but only where considerable wasting has occurred. In particular muscular dystrophies, however (congenital myotonia, acquired myotonia, myotonic dystrophy), percussion evokes a sustained local contraction. This is called percussion myotonia. In tetany, percussion of the facial nerve in the parotid region causes a twitch in the orbicularis (Chvostek's sign), but this seldom occurs with other nerves or from direct percussion of the muscle. Contraction of muscles evoked by occlusion of the circulation (Trousseau's sign) is limited to tetany. More accurate testing of the excitability of muscle and nerve is afforded by electrical testing.

Fatigue increases all kinds of muscular weakness, but only in myasthenia gravis is actual paralysis induced by use of the muscles. The patient will complain not of feeling tired or of aching muscles, but of extreme weakness after exercise. When severe, the weakness is present on awakening, without exercise, and may persist for days or weeks at a time. It is extremely unusual for the limb muscles to be involved without ptosis, weakness in extraocular muscles, or masseters, and the most convincing test for myasthenic paralysis is therefore either to get the patient to look upward at the examiner's finger steadily for one minute (which should induce ptosis if the levator is affected, sometimes strabismus) or to raise the lower jaw every two seconds against resistance applied by the examiner (if the masseters are affected, great weakness will be felt after 4-10 repetitions). In the arms, similar muscular failure with use can be elicited by making the patient abduct the arm at the shoulder or extend the elbow repeatedly against resistance. Note that no pain or aching in the muscles is evoked.

The drug edrophonium (tensilon) may be used as a therapeutic test when weakness has been noted by some particular test. The effort required for elicitation of weakness is documented, and the patient is then given 2 mg. of tensilon intravenously. If there is no untoward reaction, 8 mg. more is given. In a matter of seconds to a minute, myasthenic weakness should be reversed. While the test is frequently positive in myasthenia, the response may be absent or only equivocally positive in some patients. A false positive result is also seen rarely in other muscular disorders.

*Incoordination.* This is best demonstrated by a series of tests. The finger-nose-finger test and the heel-knee test show action (intention) tremors. Note especially, in tremors of cerebellar origin, the rhythmical tremor at right angles to the line of movement and overshooting the object, compared with the irregular unsteadiness of sensory ataxia. Then proceed to alternating movement tests, such as alternating pronation-supination (note if he fixes the elbow in doing this) and patting the observer's hand. Does his repetitive movement become held up by a conflict between the rhythms of voluntary movement and of tremor?

Rhythmical nodding of the head, with the rhythm similar to that of nystagmus or of action tremor of the limbs, is seen when cerebellar ataxia affects the neck muscles and is called titubation or static tremor. It may affect the entire vertebral column. Some slight degree of muscular contraction must be present, and no tremor is seen on complete relaxation.

Since some kinds of ataxia affect the bilateral muscles of the trunk much more than the limbs, it is important to examine the patient's gait and stance in your tests for coordination. Reeling gait is noted under general impressions, as discussed earlier. Irregular, stamping, or high-stepping movements in walking will be noted again under coordination of the legs. Lack of natural swinging of an arm, or unusual posture, such as abduction of one arm in walking, and what are called "associated movements," such as involuntary grasping in one hand when the other grasps strongly, should be noted under coordination of the arms.

*Resistance to passive movement.* The postural tone in each limb is then appraised. Here you will note any undue resistance of the muscles to passive lengthening and which groups of muscles are affected. The resistance usually accompanying damage to the corticospinal system (spasticity) has a "clasp-knife" character. The resistance is greatest soon after passive stretch begins and gives away relatively suddenly as passive stretch is persisted in. The resistance is greater the more rapidly the passive movement is made. Spasticity affects the flexors of fingers, wrist, and elbow, and to a lesser extent the extensors of elbow and adductors of shoulder, in the arm. In the leg, spasticity affects extensors of hip and knee and plantar flexors of the ankle. It is constant from hour to hour but varies from day to day. It is slight in degree for the first 2 to 4 weeks after a sudden and severe lesion and is then felt in gentle manipulation of the wrist. Do not call every kind of resistance to passive movement "spasticity." If there is inconsistent resistance simply note it as such, for it is probably related to voluntary or involuntary postures more complex than spasticity. True spasticity should be associated with increased tendon reflexes. If the spasticity is intense, the muscle may be too contracted to show a tendon reflex, which may then be revealed only when the muscle is shortened as much as possible.

Spasticity is best estimated by passive manipulation, with the patient instructed to relax as much as possible. Passive shaking of a limb, sudden passive lifting of one thigh and observation of the sagging of the leg, and such procedures may assist in estimating the presence of slight degrees of spasticity, but it is important to make sure that the patient relaxes fully. Slight spasticity can be well estimated, when its perception during manipulation is difficult, by watching the slowing it causes in alternating movement and the slowing of flexion of the hip joints in walking or running.

The rigidity of extrapyramidal disease is characterized by its more constant resistance throughout a passive manipulation (i.e., the clasp-knife feature is lacking). It is more truly plastic and affects both flexion and extension at all joints. When extrapyramidal tremor is present, even in very slight degree, the resistance to passive movement is felt to give in a series of small regular jerks (cogwheel rigidity). This is best felt by very gentle manipulation of the wrist. Confirmation of extrapyramidal type of rigidity is seen in the patient's ability to maintain awkward postures of the body (e.g., leaning slightly forward or keeping the head slightly raised from the pillow) without discomfort, and in the rarity of small associated movements such as blinking, movements of facial expression (thus resulting in the staring masklike appearance), the lack of small, continual readjustments of posture which characterize the behavior of a normal person, and the lack of arm swinging in walking.

When more intense, this extrapyramidal rigidity becomes fixed, or relatively fixed, dystonia. This is essentially an abnormal attitude. Any passive movement of the limb to alter the attitude (for example to overcome the dystonic clenched fist, inverted foot, flexed hip, or torticollic spasm of the neck) encounters a more springy type of resistance than is found in spasticity or rigidity, tending to increase with increased displacement. The part tends to fly back to the original posture when released.

Resistance to passive movement is also found in the abnormal attitudes of the limbs of patients in stuporous or comatose states, especially decorticate and decerebrate attitudes associated with tentorial herniation. The paralyzed limb is commonly flaccid, and the abnormal posture in the sound limbs reflects more transient disorder of motor function than do spasticity, rigidity, or dystonia. Such a posture is then usually a transient variant of decorticate attitude (flexed arms with pronation, extended legs) or decerebrate rigidity (extension of all limbs). If there is rigidity that has inconsistencies, such as variation from moment to moment, hysteria must be suspected. If the rigidity is associated with pain on manipulation, either hysteria or some local painful lesion should be considered. If there is firm fixed limitation of the degree of passive movement, then either muscle is permanently shortened (contracture) or the condition of the joint merits special inquiry.

Lack of muscular tone (hypotonia) is also estimated by passive manipulation, but as the natural degree of muscular tone is slight, hypotonia is best estimated by carefully watching the movements of the joints when the relaxed limb is shaken or suddenly displaced. Is the wrist unduly free when the observer takes the forearm and passively shakes it? Does the outstretched arm swing unduly freely when suddenly knocked aside by the examiner? Another method is to see how rapidly the movement is checked when the limb is thrown violently into unexpected movement. In estimating this, you may suddenly throw the patient's hand toward his face, or having made him pull hard, with semiflexed elbow, against your hand, you suddenly let go (rebound phenomenon). The hypotonic limb has an unnatural "fling" or lack of braking action. Hypotonia also affects in some degree the limits of passive movements of joints, so that the wrist can be dorsiflexed further than normal, and the patient's attempt to hold the hand fully extended results in overextension of the metacarpophalangeal joints (the choreic hand).

It must be emphasized that the most reliable estimation of change in tone is the resistance to passive manipulation of the limb, and tests such as those mentioned above are merely confirmatory.

If weakness or paralysis of flaccid type is present, it is well to ask yourself at this stage if it corresponds to the distribution of segmental nerve roots or has an upper level corresponding to the innervation of one nerve root, or on the other hand if it corresponds to the distribution of a peripheral nerve or a group of such nerves. A list of the segmental supplies of the chief muscle groups is given in Table 1. The general plan of innervation by the major peripheral nerves should be familiar to you.

It is possible that the longest nerves are affected most, giving a weakness which is the more severe the more distal a muscle is from the spinal cord. Recheck the relative strengths of muscles to find if the weakness conforms to any of these types.

If spasticity is present, where is its upper level? What is the most rostral segment that is affected? Check this against any segmental level of sensory disorder.

*Involuntary movements.* Last, note any involuntary movements that are present. They are usually seen when the limbs are at rest, as for example the rhythmical tremor of Parkinsonism, but may be more obvious in movement, as is chorea.

The tremor of Parkinsonism has a characteristic regular rhythm, seen best in the rhythmical alternating flexion-extension of the fingers with adduction-abduction of thumb (pill-rolling tremor), and tremor of the lips and of the eyelids when lightly closed. When severe, the tremor involves the wrist and ankle, elbow and hip. It is lessened or halted by movement but reasserts itself in the new posture when the movement is complete (cerebellar tremor, in contrast, is a tremor of movement and involves proximal joints). In complete relaxation the Parkinsonian tremor ceases, but the patient has the greatest difficulty in relaxing to this extent, maintaining some mild attitudinal contraction in almost all states except deep sleep.

Senile tremor is a less constant rhythmical tremor of the fingers, sometimes of the wrist, more obvious in the outstretched hands than at rest, slightly increased by movement, and associated with a side-to-side tremor of the head. Familial tremor most commonly takes the form of a fairly rapid tremor of the fingers of the outstretched hands, absent at rest, and usually lessened greatly by movement. Only with Parkinsonism is there associated plastic rigidity. Hysterical tremor tends to involve the whole limb or whole body and is greatly worsened by any attempt to control the movement. In hepatic disorders a tendency of the outstretched hands to flap rhythmically at the wrists (liver flap, asterixis) may appear. A similar flapping tremor at wrists and shoulders (wing beating) is associated with hepatolenticular degeneration (Wilson's disease).

Less rhythmical involuntary movements are grouped into myoclonus, athetosis, or chorea, according to their type and distribution. Myoclonus is a sudden brief jerk or contraction of a muscle or muscle group. It can occur as multiple irregular coarse twitchings of any muscle in some types of encephalitis (herpes, inclusion-body encephalitis), and then is associated with an occasional jerk of spinal muscles. A sudden flexion of one or both arms, irregularly repeated, is another variant. Myoclonus may be associated with epilepsy but is not itself epileptic. Epileptic twitching takes the form of a slowly repeated series of brief spasms in muscles that have just passed through the tonic phase of convulsion. A rhythmical instability of the palate resulting from some types of damage to the brain stem is called palatal myoclonus.

Athetosis is essentially an instability of posture. It is most commonly seen in the hand, which swings from a widely extended position, usually with supination, to a tightly flexed pronated posture, the thumb usually being strongly adducted and trapped by the tightly flexed fingers. When spasticity is present, alternation between these two postures is slow and deliberate, the fingers opening and closing one by one. When there is no associated spasticity, the hand opens and closes rapidly but irregularly, the whole cycle taking 1 to 5 seconds. Athetosis commonly complicates hemiplegia dating from infancy and is often partial in degree, the fingers tending to postural instability but not making full swings. Sometimes more rapid jerks are superimposed on an athetotic posture of the hand (choreoathetosis). When athetosis is generalized (double athetosis) as a result of degenerative disease of the basal ganglia, the whole arm may flex and extend, the lips and tongue be distorted by alternating protrusions and retractions, and the toes and foot fluctuate between extension and flexion-inversion.

In Huntington's chorea the same abnormal postures of athetosis are seen, but in fluid and irregular sequence and associated with many partial and conflicting movements, so that some fingers may flex while others are opening, for example. A sweeping side-to-side movement of the head associated with a grimace is common. All movements are more obvious as the patient walks, the hesitations in gait, athetoid movements of the hands, and grimaces then providing the "dance" that gave the name chorea.

In Sydenham's chorea the most obvious abnormality is sudden lapses of contraction. When the hands are outstretched, one or another finger flexes momentarily, or the wrist or the whole arm drops for a moment and is then replaced. The facial expression is momentarily interrupted by a twitch. The lapses are irregular in type and recurrence, so that the movement is unpredictable. Any willed movement is liable to similar interruption, as may be felt if the patient is asked to maintain a steady grasp of the observer's hand. The movements most commonly affect the limbs and face on one side, but when severe they become generalized and may then be associated with active flinging movements of a whole limb and with interruptions of respiration. The affected limbs are hypotonic, and the arms tend to pronate when held out or above the head.

Hemiballismus is a flinging movement of the whole arm at the shoulders with associated restless flexions and extensions at the hip. There is often an associated irregular opening and closing of the hand (posthemiplegic chorea).

Tics, or "nervous habits," are movements that are stereotyped; that is, the movement is repeated at irregular intervals in precisely the same form. The patient can suppress the movement for a time but has an increasing feeling of need to make it, so that sooner or later the movement recurs. He can also make the movement at will. The movement can take any form, such as blinking the eyes, shrugging one shoulder, expiring noisily with a cough, twitching the body, each such movement being peculiar to the patient. One patient may have several tics, each of which is repeated at irregular intervals. Tics are distinguished from mannerisms only by the degree to which they are unusual and become a source of embarrassment to the individual.

## Reflexes

The reflexes serve as sensitive indicators of the state of the nervous center and its afferent pathway.

The pupillary, corneal, and palatal reflexes have been dealt with under cranial nerves.

The tendon reflexes, abdominal reflexes, and the plantar responses should be examined as a routine, and the anal and bulbocavernous reflexes in addition in all suspected conus or cauda equina lesions or cases of sphincteric disturbances.

*Tendon reflexes.* For elicitation of the tendon reflexes,

adequate relaxation on the part of the patient is essential. A certain mild degree of passive tension on the muscle is also necessary; especially in the case of the radial (supinator) and ankle jerks, the observer may have to vary the tension on the muscle by manipulating the joint before being certain the jerk is unobtainable. If the patient is not completely relaxed it is helpful to engage his attention in some other occupation such as pulling on one hand with the other (reinforcement). In addition he might be instructed to give an extra pull on his hands just as the observer strikes.

Good relaxation of the tendo Achillis is obtained if the patient kneels on a chair. When the patient is lying down, the most advantageous position for eliciting the ankle jerk is with the thigh externally rotated, the knee semiflexed, and the ankle a little inverted. The plantar response can conveniently be elicited with the foot in the same position, although if there is some doubt as to the outcome the leg should be extended fully.

In eliciting the triceps jerk it is important to disregard the small direct contraction of those muscles directly percussed by the hammer, for most muscles will contract if directly percussed. If the muscle is extremely spastic the tendon jerk, though present, may be submerged by contraction (the muscle fibers being already contracted). The jerk is normally present in only a part of each muscle, and in a purely muscular disease such as myopathy the jerk may be lost in quadriceps through wasting of the vastus internus, though the power of contraction of the remainder is still of fair degree. Lastly, a small percentage of otherwise normal people have never possessed tendon reflexes (congenital areflexia).

A slight finger jerk is normally present and is of value only when its briskness on one side confirms a suspicion of one-sided increase in the arm jerks. A flick of the patient's finger-nail has the same effect in providing a sudden stretch of the flexor tendon and causing a sudden flexion response in all fingers (Hoffmann's sign). Likewise, a slight jaw jerk (a light downward tap on the chin with the mouth half open) is some-times normally present, and only when there is a brisk re-sponse is there evidence that an upper motoneuron lesion exists, confirmed if a tap of the examiner's finger stretching a facial muscle elicits a facial jerk.

*Abdominal reflexes.* The abdominal reflexes are chiefly of use when there is a one-sided difference, or when they are lost below a certain level which coincides with other evidence of the disturbance at that segment. The upper abdominal re-flexes are the most sensitive and are obtained by light stroking from the lower ribs over the epigastrium. Abdominal dis-tension, full bladder, or menstruation also temporarily abolish the reflexes, so that bilateral loss is of value only as a confirmation of other evidence of upper motor neuron lesion.

*Plantar response.* The plantar response is the most valu-able physical sign in the nervous system. The response is not a simple reflex but is the outcome of two, probably three, reflex effects, the balance of which is disturbed by damage to motor centers in the brain or their pathways in the spinal cord. The normal response is a slow, deliberate plantar flexion of the great toe, and for clinical purposes movement at the meta-tarsophalangeal joint should alone be observed. The stimulus may be nociceptive, tactile, or proprioceptive, but the most suitable is a light stroking movement by an object with blunt pointed end, such as a key, for painful stimulation induces a voluntary movement which confuses the outcome. Proprio-ceptive stimuli have a high threshold and are not so reliable. The site of stimulation is the outer border of the sole of the foot, for as the abnormal reflex appears it can first be obtained here (at a time when the response from the inner border is still flexor), and the receptive area later spreads to the rest of the foot. The reflex may be obtained from any part of the lower limb, or even the abdominal wall when reflex activity is fully exaggerated.

For the elicitation of the plantar response the leg should be relaxed as much as possible, the foot warm, and the stimulating stroke deliberate from heel to the ball of the great toe. If there is dorsiflexion of the ankle or withdrawal of the limb, reduce the intensity of stimulus to get movement of the toe alone if possible.

The abnormal reflex is a dorsiflexion, often quick, at the metatarsophalangeal joint. Only practice in eliciting the reflex will enable the observer to make critical judgment in cases where the outcome is equivocal. Attempts to decide a doubtful response on the basis of other procedures such as those of Oppenheim, Gordon, or Rossolimo are not recommended.* The plantar response may be absent owing to interference with its reflex arc (damage to sacral segments, roots, or nerves).

Occasionally, as a result of old spinal cord damage, ankle clonus is present when the plantar response has again become flexor. In progressive lesions it is of later appearance than other signs and is confirmatory of exaggeration of the ankle jerk. For its elicitation it is important to have the ankle relaxed as much as possible, knee semiflexed, and to make passive dorsiflexion suddenly but not too forcibly. False ankle clonus sometimes occurs in nervous people with tense

*Descriptions of these and other reflex signs can be found in Department of Neurology, Mayo Clinic and Foundations, *Clinical Examinations in Neurology*, 4th ed. (Philadelphia: W. B. Saunders, 1976).

muscles and brisk jerks, and the gait is not then spastic. If during the clonus the observer painfully overflexes the patient's great toe, true clonus stops momentarily while false clonus is increased, but this is not a completely reliable differentiation.

*Anal reflex.* The superficial anal reflex is a contraction of the levator ani and associated perineal muscles when a pin is drawn along the sacral skin on either side of the anus. It is lost following damage to the third or fourth sacral segments of spinal cord or their nerve roots.

A sudden softening of the anal sphincter on insertion of the examiner's finger followed by further gaping on withdrawal is described as the internal anal reflex, but is not a true reflex. It is the normal reaction of the internal anal sphincter and is not apparent in the normal patient, owing to the postural contraction of the striped external anal sphincter, which grasps the finger gently. The softening is therefore a sign of loss of innervation of the external sphincter (S3, 4).

Owing to confusion in terminology, it is therefore wise to describe these responses or their lack in terms of what you observe, rather than to say "anal reflex positive" or "present." In the same say the minus sign ($-$) should not be used, because of its ambiguity. Use instead 0 for absent, and diminished or dimin. for lessened.

To conclude, the only absolute reflex sign is the plantar response. Briskness or sluggishness of tendon jerks or abdominal reflexes is only of significance in relation to other evidence or when one-sided.

When damage to conducting pathways is sudden and severe, all reflex activity below the lesion may for some days be depressed (spinal shock). The tendon jerks then gradually become hyperactive, and the plantar response progressively more abnormal. In complete spinal transection a weak flexor movement of the great toe may be found in the first week. This is a small reflex from the sacral segments and is soon overcome by the more intense dorsiflexion which is part of the withdrawal reflex (the true Babinski phenomenon).

*Sphincteric reflexes.* The sphincters show a special type of reflex function. The internal vesical sphincter is an integral part of the bladder mechanism, which always works as a whole except when there is structural deformity of the bladder neck.

The filling and emptying of the bladder is an automatic process by which distension beyond a certain degree evokes contraction waves in the bladder. These rise in intensity to reach a mass contraction which empties the contents. In the normal person this reaction is postponed by higher centers, at first subconsciously, and when more intense, consciously, until a convenient time. Voluntary micturition is a round-about process of willed relaxation of this inhibition. If micturition has been postponed, any sudden abolition of cerebral function (sudden unconsciousness) will abolish the inhibitory restraint and cause micturition. Thus occurs the involuntary incontinence of epilepsy.

The spincter may be regarded as doing exactly the opposite of what the bladder muscle does (contraction of detrusor with relaxation of sphincter, and vice versa) owing to a simple nervous arrangement in the vesical plexus (as in the normal pylorus).

The reaction of the bladder to a nervous lesion may therefore be regarded solely in the light of what happens to the bladder wall (detrusor). Sudden interruption of nervous pathways connecting the higher centers with the vesical neurons in the spinal cord in the second and third sacral segments results in transitory depression of their reflex function (spinal shock), and the reflex activity of micturition is lost. The detrusor is then atonic and not responsive to stretch, just as the voluntary muscles are flaccid in that stage. The bladder becomes very distended, and unless relieved there is severe damage to the mucosa (hemorrhagic cystitis). If this is avoided, reaction to stretch slowly begins to recover from spinal shock, and in a few days the detrusor begins to contract a little when stretched. Soon larger contractions appear, and the relaxations of the sphincter which automatically accompany them are sufficient to allow the bladder to empty itself of some of its contents. Later, with full reflex activity, the contractions may empty the bladder completely and may be facilitated by any change in abdominal pressure (cough, movement) or by sensory stimulation of the limbs or perineum (full reflex micturition).

With slowly advancing cord or bilateral brain lesions, the reflex hyperactivity increases as voluntary restraint is being lessened, and the intermediate stages—frequency, urgency with some control and periodic incontinence—progress to full incontinence. The frequency, urgency, and inability to restrain will be described by the patient.

Sudden damage to the sacral segments themselves or to the nerve roots (S2 and S3) connecting them to the pelvic nerve also throws the bladder wall into atony, with corresponding complete retention of urine (i.e., the inevitable inverse hypertonia of the internal sphincter). In time the detrusor regains some reaction to stretch, but this is feeble in degree and is seldom, except in children, able to cause efficient micturition. The corresponding slight loosening of the sphincter, however, allows these patients to void urine by abdominal straining (the abdominal segmental innervation is above the lesion). The resulting periodic dribbling is called "automatic micturition" and is independent of the central nervous system. It is sometimes seen as a result of spina bifida affecting the cauda equina. More usually there is retention of urine with dribbling micturition because the detrusor remains weak. When a cauda equina lesion develops slowly, micturition becomes more and more difficult, the bladder more and more trabeculated from the distension. The patient will describe his increasing difficulty, dribbling stream, and inability to complete micturition.

Sacral cord or root disease therefore diminishes bladder reflex function just as the ankle jerks served by the first and second sacral segments are diminished and then lost. Interference with the afferent side of the reflex arc acts in just the same way, so that there is no essential difference between the tabetic bladder and the cauda equina bladder. The function of the sympathetic (hypogastric nerve) innervation is disregarded in the interpretation of nervous disorders of micturition (it is related to ejaculation).

The mechanism of the anal sphincter is affected in exactly the same way, so that upper motor neuron lesions will cause active massive incontinence, and lower motor lesions will cause passive rectal distension with leaking sphincter. These states are seen, however, only with fluid feces, and usually both types become constipated. In both, the sphincter is normally closed but easily loosened by stimulation (see anal reflex, above).

## Sensation

It is manifestly unnecessary to test every small part of the skin surface with every modality of sensation in every patient.

It is, however, advisable to test each of the four extremities for changes in sensation to pin prick, and for position sense in the joints of fingers and toes as a routine, for this will sometimes pick up a type of change in sensation of which the patient is not aware.

For the other kinds of testing of sensation there are certain well-defined indications:

1. Any complaint or admission of numbness, pins and needles, tingling, coldness, or pain should lead to careful test of sensation for touch, pain, heat and cold, position sense, and vibration sense in the part concerned.

2. The finding of localized atrophy or weakness should prompt a search for sensory loss in corresponding nerves or nerve roots.

3. The presence of ataxia should always lead to careful estimation of position and vibration sense.

4. Trophic changes, especially painless ulcers, blisters, and joint affections, should lead to careful testing for loss of pain sense.

5. When a cerebral lesion is suspected, discriminative sensation (position sense, two-point) should be estimated on the two sides.

*Touch.* This is best tested with a small wisp of cotton fiber twisted so as to leave only a few fibers at its tip. Care must be taken to avoid hairs in critical testing, for the hair follicle is a coarse receptor. Allowance must be made for the thicker skin on the palm and sole. For stronger stimulation, light strokes may be employed. If the cooperation of the patient is doubted, ask him to close his eyes and indicate each touch.

*Pain.* The sense of pain is estimated by pin prick, and the pricks should be even and not too rapid (about one a second). If there is an area of lack of response or of blunted sensation, define it by proceeding from the region of blunting in various directions, marking the point of reaching normal sensation with a fiber tip pen or marker. It is important to realize that in many kinds of sensory loss the border is not sharp and is a zone of graduated impairment. Therefore deeper, heavier pin pricks will show a smaller area of loss than will a series of light pin pricks. Very slight changes can be defined in a cooperative patient by getting him to indicate the change in sensation when a pin point is lightly dragged over the skin. When an area of sensory loss is charted, it may be considered whether it is consistent with an area of segmental skin innervation (see Chart 1, giving approximate segmental areas), or with the pattern supplied by any peripheral nerve or nerve group (Charts 2 and 3). If there is loss or diminution of sensation below a particular level, check the two sides to see if they are the same. The area may correspond to a zone or band of several segments, or may be the result of heaviest affection of the longest fibers, as in some kinds of neuritis. These things are most easily determined for sensation to pin prick, and other sensation is then reexamined to find if the pattern of loss is the same for all forms or affects each differently (dissociated sensory loss).

The area of involvement of a lightly moving tactile touch is especially sensitive in defining peripheral nerve sensory distributions, and on occasion spinal levels can best be delineated in this fashion.

The experienced observer is on the watch for altered pilomotor reactions, sweating, and temperature and color of the skin with which to confirm his findings.

Inconsistency in the patient's replies should always lead to suspicion of suggestion and cause one to devise other means of testing sensation (i.e., is there astereognosis or incoordina-

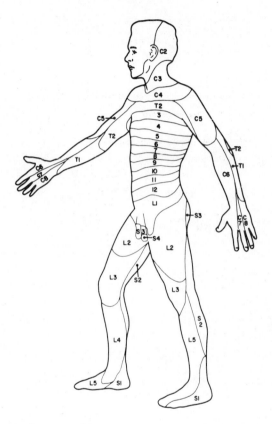

Chart 1. Segmental innervation of the skin (after Foerster). There is extensive overlap of innervation of skin by nerve roots, so the loss of sensation is far less than the whole root territory. (Reproduced by permission, from Webb Haymaker and Barnes Woodhall, *Peripheral Nerve Injuries* (Philadelphia, W. B. Saunders, 1945).

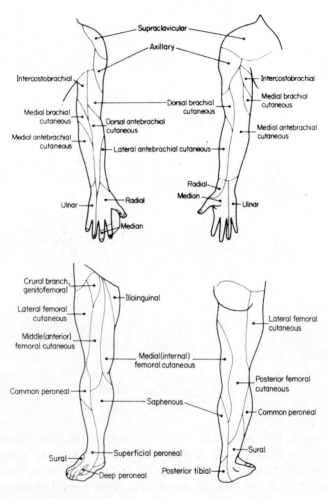

Chart 2. Cutaneous nerve distribution over the arms and legs.

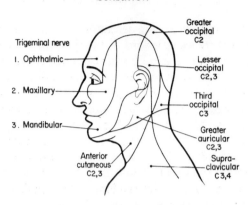

Chart 3. Cutaneous nerve distribution over the head and neck.

tion commensurate with the supposed sensory loss, or is the sensory loss changed by strong countersuggestion?).

It is very easy for sensory loss to be suggested to an anxious patient by the very fact that it is being tested. This usually begins by the patient making too much of some small difference. If the patient states there is some small difference between one side and the other, attempt to decide how much difference there is by giving different intensities of pin prick. It is usually possible to break through the early stages of suggested analgesia by repeated painful pin prick.

In special forms of sensory loss (e.g., in syringomyelia) the presence of acute touch sensation enables the patient to say "It's sharp," though he may perceive no pain. If you suspect that this is happening, ask him to indicate when the prick hurts him. Observation of the amount of wincing produced by equivalent pricks in different areas also gives a more objective finding.

Raised threshold of pain sensation with overreaction is a common occurrence in lesions of the spinothalamic pathway and sometimes in cerebral cortical lesions. Single pricks at long intervals are then not appreciated or are felt as dulled. More rapidly repeated pricking is suddenly felt as intensely painful, more painful than on the normal side. A single severe prick may also have abnormally prolonged tingling.

*Heat and cold.* This sense should be tested with tubes of hot and cold water. The area of loss to sensation to heat is usually larger than that of loss to cold. The two tubes are touched against the skin at random and the patient asked to indicate the temperature changes. When loss is found, move the tube along the skin until change occurs. Chart the areas of loss with oblique lines, obliquity one way for heat, another for cold.

*Position.* In testing sense of position, it is necessary to hold both segments at the joint firmly to prevent difference of cutaneous contact from indicating the movement at the joint. The degree of movement should be varied in each movement, for loss of ability to recognize large movements occurs only when the damage to position sense is severe. In spinal diseases the loss of sense of position is usually maximal in the toes and fingers, but in some kinds of polyneuritis it may affect the proximal joints and not the distal, thus causing an ataxia of gait without loss of sense of position in the great toe. To demonstrate this, get the patient to close his eyes and then manipulate his leg to some extreme angle and ask him to point to where he thinks his great toe is.

*Vibration.* The sense of vibration is a variety of deep cutaneous sensation, a rapid alteration of pressure sense. It is felt best over any hard resistance and thus usually over bony prominences, though it can be felt equally well by loose skin, for example the abdominal wall, if a fold of skin is held between the tuning fork and some hard object. A tuning fork with low rate of vibration (128 p.s.) should be used, and the heavier the better. For exact work, a fork with an attachment indicating a standard amplitude of vibration is used and the time to cessation of sensation measured. For ordinary clinical purposes it is sufficient to record less or diminution of the sensation. Be sure that the patient understands that it is the vibration (buzzing) and not the pressure that he is expected to feel. Loss of vibration sense is sometimes more severe than loss of position (e.g., in combined system disease), sometimes the reverse (multiple sclerosis), but both types of sensation are usually affected together in some degree except in cortical lesions (see below). Vibration sense is diminished in advancing age and impaired by adiposity.

*Discriminative sensation.** Damage to the sensory mechanism above the level of the thalamus affects the ability to make certain sensory discriminations. The most obvious and most easily tested of these is the ability to appreciate joint movement. Thus position sense may be lost and ataxia may occur, without loss of vibration sense, from parietal cortical lesion. When this occurs there should also be some loss of ability to discriminate two points from one point. A compass with blunt tips is used for this, and the distance apart is adjusted according to the normal threshold of the part tested (e.g., 3 mm. at tip of finger, 1 cm. for palm of hand, 4 to 7 cms. on the body surface). Begin on the supposed normal side

*For further details of tests for discriminative sensation, see Henry Head, *Studies in Neurology*, vol. 1 (Oxford: Oxford University Press, 1920), ch. 2; Henry Head and Gordon Holmes, "Sensory Disturbances from Cerebral Lesions," *Brain* 34 (1911-12): 102; and Gordon Holmes, *Brain* 50 (1917): 413.

and satisfy yourself that the patient can discriminate between a light pressure for two or three seconds (the exact time does not matter) of one point and of two points. Then test the abnormal side. Record the result in two columns (one point and two points), indicating a correct answer by a stroke and incorrect by a cross.

The same loss of sensation can be shown more easily but not so accurately by writing numbers with a blunt object on the patient's skin while his eyes are closed and getting him to indicate what the number was.

With this type of sensory loss there is also a difficulty in localization of points touched (charted by marking the point touched with a cross on a diagram of the part and connecting this by a line to an arrow head showing where the patient thought he was touched). Ability to discriminate between different degrees of temperature and of pain, and different weights, may be affected but is more difficult to test without special apparatus.

The ability to assess the texture and exact shape of an object requires a complex sensory differentiation. When there is loss of two-point discrimination there is usually also loss of ability to recognize the form of an object placed in the hand (key, coin, ring, etc.). This is often loosely called astereognosis, but it is better to call it lack of recognition of shape and form.

True astereognosis is by definition a defect at a high level, a lack of perception of the nature of an object felt, the primary sense data being intact. It is dependent upon loss of spatial summation and is a defect in the parietal lobe function in perception. In actuality some impairment of tactile discrimination is usually present. Lack of recognition of form, however, may be present in cord (dorsal column) and medullary lesions and is then dependent upon the more elementary disorder of postural and tactile sense.

Of the various kinds of loss of sensory discrimination, sense of position and of two-point discrimination are always affected as well as the others, and being easier to test are usually alone investigated. Stereognosis is less delicate but often used. It should be noted that some forms of parietal lesion affect summation of pain and temperature sensation, often with predominantly radial or ulnar distribution, so that it is not sufficient to test, for instance, just the index finger.

Sensation is a subjective phenomenon. The patient may unconsciously edit such information as you derive from sensory testing. If all the abnormal findings are sensory, review them with an eye to the possibility that they have been suggested by examination and are not the result of disease. Beware of reliance on sensory change unaccompanied by any complaint such as numbness, paresthesia, or ataxia. In doubtful cases, confirmation of sensory disturbance can be obtained from sweating tests, for in peripheral nerve lesions and also some types of central lesion the sympathetic supply suffers disorder over a similar area (see under Special Investigations).

### Tenderness, Palpation, and Tests of Neuromuscular Structures

The patient's complaint of pain naturally leads the physician to palpate local structures for tenderness. Since pain from nervous lesions is commonly referred to the periphery, it is necessary to explore the length of the neurons leading from the part complained of. The nerve roots entering the spinal cord are not directly accessible to palpation, but if the

damage is located at this point, movement of the corresponding region of the spine is limited by pain which should approximate that complained of. Note any limitation discovered
and the nature of any pain complained of during passive
movements of the head and active movements to the extremes
of flexion, extension, and torsion of the spine.

When the knees are maintained in full extension and the
hips are flexed, the sciatic nerve trunk normally makes a
slight traction on the sciatic plexus and nerve roots. In sci-
atica, trauma to the nerve or roots, damage to the plexus, or
compression of the roots, the degree to which the examiner
can raise the patient's straight leg from the bed or couch illus-
trates the degree of this limitation. Thus it may be recorded
"straight leg raising limited to 45° on the right, 90° on the
left side." The presence of such limitation is called Lasègue's
sign. The movement should be made slowly, for severe pain
may be induced by sudden movement.

In meningitis, tenderness of the nerve roots also results,
and the above sign is positive. It is traditionally elicited by
first flexing the hip with knee flexed, and then extending the
knee passively. Limitation is Kernig's sign. The mechanism is,
however, the same as in Lasègue's sign and may be expressed
quantitatively in that way. In meningitis or meningeal reaction, the corresponding limitation of neck movement due to
tenderness of the cervical nerve roots and dura is more intense, occurs earlier, and is more reliable than Kernig's sign.
This is demonstrated by resistance to passive flexion of the
neck and is termed neck rigidity. Some associated flexion of
the lower limbs as full flexion is reached is called Brudzinski's
sign, but is not of great value, as it appears only when meningeal irritation is severe.

Tenderness of the muscles accompanies some forms of

neuritis but is not always present. It also appears in poly-myositis and with some forms of hyperesthesia, as in com-bined system disease.

In some forms of neuritis (brachial neuritis, true sciatic neuritis) a widespread fibrositis may accompany or precede the involvement of nerve trunks. Then exquisitely tender points may be located along the vertebral border or over the spine of the scapula or in the gluteal muscles and are con-firmatory of fibrositis. In chronic fibrositic neuritis in the hand, the nerve trunks in the palm are tender, and in trau-matic ulnar neuritis the tender neuroma can be felt in the un-usually shallow groove at the elbow.

In persistent constant unilateral headache, tenderness of the skull should always be searched for, and rarely either bony abnormality or a tender swollen artery (temporal arter-itis) may be found.

When pain is referred to the limbs, or unexplained wasting of muscles around a joint occurs, the possibility of arthritis should be examined. This is especially important in the hip and shoulder joints, where the pain may be referred some distance and yet be reproduced by simple external rotation or abduction tests. If pain is produced by manipulation at any joint, ask the patient whether the pain is the same as that of which he complains.

Tenderness in the sacroiliac joints is often tested by com-pressing the iliac crests. A better test is to have the patient lie face down, then you press firmly on the sacrum with one hand to steady the pelvis, and with the other under the knee raise the thigh until the hip joint is strained in full retro-flexion. This should cause pain on the affected side. Lumbar vertebral disorder and affection of the hip joint should be separately excluded.

Examination of the extracerebral blood vessels is ordinarily performed in all patients. The carotid arteries should be auscultated for bruits, especially for bruits which are heard from the level of the bifurcation (about opposite the larynx) and above. Bruits may also be heard over the subclavian artery in the supraclavicular fossa. It is often difficult to decide, in patients with systolic murmurs at the cardiac base, if the bruit heard in the neck is this same murmur or an independent one.

Palpation of the force of the carotid pulse in the neck is usually unreliable. In patients with common carotid occlusion, the preauricular pulse (a branch of the external carotid) is reduced or absent. The supraorbital pulse at the upper rim of the orbit reflects the continuation of the internal carotid-ophthalmic flow. Occasionally one can demonstrate that this pulse disappears when the preauricular is compressed with one's finger, thereby showing reduction in internal carotid flow, presumably owing to stenosis.

### Deformity or Limitation of Range of Movement

The skull should be palpated in all cases of epilepsy and in any suspected cerebral involvement. Though a positive finding is rare, it is well worth the trouble taken. Old depressed fracture, recent erosion, nodular deformity, old burrholes from a previous subdural exploration or craniotomy, and general asymmetry are to be looked for. This can conveniently be combined with auscultation over the vertex and temples for bruits.

In all cases of suspected root pain or of affection of the spinal cord, the movements of the spine should be watched, and felt with the flat of the hand, during flexion and extension. Any rigidity of the spine is noted. This may be limited to one region, for example, if the patient holds the lumbar spine stiffly straight while overflexing the thoracic spine. Learning to palpate the paravertebral muscles may be useful, especially if there is segmental spasm.

Malalignment or any undue prominence of the spinal processes is noted. The spines may be percussed with a percussion hammer, or better, one of the examiner's hands may be laid flat on the suspected region, the other closed into a fist and thumped on the first to elicit local tenderness, which may be due either to a diseased vertebra or to jamming of structures in the vertebral or root canal.

Limitation of movement in other joints is noted. Does mannipulation of the related joint reproduce the pain of which the patient complains?

## Aphasia

This is a difficult area for the beginning student to master, partly because one naturally assumes that the language one hears is representative of good, normal function, and it takes a practiced ear to listen to speech on two levels, both for its desired communication and also for errors or deficits in the speech itself.

Patients who are being evaluated for language disturbance should first be evaluated for level of consciousness and full attention. The level of consciousness clearly dominates the language output, because language is one of the most obvious cognitive and intellectual functions, and its integrity is drastically altered by states that produce stupor or deficit in awareness. Patients who are confused typically have language disturbance along with other aspects of cognitive disorder.

Attention may be altered in a patient who is normally alert. The most common example of this is the so-called acute confusional state, also known as toxic encephalopathy or toxic delirium. With this condition the patient is severely inattentive and produces very incoherent speech which drifts away from the point of beginning. He may often demonstrate markedly impaired memory and orientation. Many patients who are confused also have hallucinations, agitation, and marked degrees of cognitive disorder. Confusional state is an important behavior pattern to recognize, because it usually represents a metabolic imbalance, a toxic reaction to drugs or sepsis, or medical illness in general. The language disturbance may be the most apparent and may be the initial sign that the patient is in fact confused. Only with further testing can it be demonstrated that the patient is severely inattentive and disoriented. See the tests for attentiveness and orientation, in particular the tests requiring serial repeated function such as serial 7 subtraction or digit retention.

If the patient has been found to be alert and attentive, his language can be usefully tested. It is well to begin this testing by listening to his spontaneous speech. If the patient does not speak freely, the examiner should ask open-ended questions, such as, "Tell me a bit about your work," or "Tell me why you are in the hospital." These will keep the patient from answering "yes" or "no" and allow sufficient speech for evaluation.

In evaluating spontaneous speech an obvious point, often immediately apparent, is whether the speech is fluent or nonfluent. A patient with nonfluent speech makes a great effort to speak, and the speech produced is sparse in amount, usually consisting chiefly of nouns without grammatical connective words; there are frequent pauses while the patient searches for a word.

Fluent aphasic speech, on the other hand, usually is characterized by a normal or even excessively rapid rate of word production. The words are often difficult to recognize, and there are many kinds of word errors, termed paraphasias. These may be neologistic (new word) paraphasias or may consist of substitutions of syllables in a word that is otherwise correct. A complete word substitution is called a verbal paraphasia. When fluent speech contains many paraphasias and is delivered at a rapid rate of speed, it is termed jargon aphasia.

During the evaluation of normal spontaneous speech, the patient can also be evaluated for the presence of dysarthria, which may be an important component of many types of nonfluent aphasia.

Comprehension of spoken speech, the next step in a careful language evaluation, is difficult to assess and is often a stumbling point for the student. Many clinicians test comprehension by asking patients to carry out specific motor commands, which works well if the patient is able to do the task. If the task is done and is sufficiently complex, one can take the results to indicate that verbal comprehension has been normal. Tests of this kind might include, "Place your left index finger on your right kneecap," or, "Show me by raising your fingers the number of the letter in the alphabet that corresponds to the first letter of your name."

Many patients who have aphasia of one type or another are unable to carry through commands of this type; nevertheless, their comprehension may be quite normal. In this case, one is observing a disorder of motor production, called apraxia, which is making the evaluation more difficult. Therefore, if the patient fails on tests of this type, he should be asked a series of questions requiring a "yes" or "no" answer, or in which he points to the correct answer. For instance, a patient could be asked, "Show me where the window is," or when shown a series of objects, he could be asked to point to the coins, the pencil, the key, and so forth. If he passes these tests, more complex questions can be asked that do not require a motor response, such as, "Do you eat breakfast before lunch?"

Repetition of spoken language is a somewhat different function from natural, spontaneous speech. In one type of aphasia, repetition is characteristically disturbed. Therefore, the patient should be asked to repeat single words or short phrases in which there are many small connecting words. The phrase, "No, ifs, ands or buts," is traditionally used, or one may ask the patient to say, "He and she and I went out." Minor errors are significant.

The ability to name objects is characteristically disturbed with practically all aphasias. In fact, it is so nonspecific a finding that many patients who have confusion or dementia rather than a specific type of aphasia may have difficulties with naming. Therefore anomia, or an anomic aphasia, is not likely to be significant in terms of cortical localization of a process. The words used for naming tests should include simple, common names, such as the parts of the body, as well as more difficult terms, such as the parts of a watch or unusual colors.

Reading ability should be tested in a patient with aphasia, and this should include having the patient read aloud fairly long paragraphs, with the examiner listening for paraphastic errors, as well as shorter sentences that test the patient's comprehension. In some instances, writing words on small cards and then asking the patient to read them may be useful. In a hospital setting it may be important to assist the patient in some ways since he may have difficulty in seeing or in following the words along the line.

Writing may be important and should be tested in a comprehensive testing for speech. A patient with nonfluent aphasia usually has a comparable disorder of writing and in a situation in which dysarthria is very severe and there is doubt whether or not an aphasia exists, writing may decide this conclusively. Rarely, patients may show a writing disorder only or may have the interesting syndrome of being able to write but not able to read what they have just written.

Aphasic syndromes that are observed in patients are typically mixtures of variable types of impairment. It is beyond the scope of this book to indicate the different types of aphasia that may exist, and interested readers are referred to other books for this knowledge. The observation that a patient is clearly and definitely aphasic is an important one to make, and the description of whether a patient has a fluent or nonfluent aphasia, normal comprehension, normal writing, and other such basic observations should also be possible for every patient with an organic cerebral disorder.

## Perceptive Disorder, Agnosia, and Apraxia

Specific syndromes may result from lesions affecting some parts of the association cortex. Frequently, considerable specialized testing is required to define these abnormalities, and the student is referred to other texts for these methods.* The abnormalities will be briefly referred to here so that their general character can be recognized.

*Neglect syndrome.* As a result of a lesion of the nondominant parietal lobe the patient may ignore the opposite (usually left) side of his body and limbs, fail to cover the left side with his clothing, fail to brush his hair on the left side, and, when

*Richard L. Strub and F. William Black, *The Mental Status Examination in Neurology* (Philadelphia: F. A. Davis, 1977).

the condition is severe, deny that the left limbs are his or that he has disability in them. It is unilateral and applies also to events and objects in the corresponding side of extrapersonal space if the lesion involves the posterior parietal lobe.

*Apraxia.* This is the inability to perform a given motor act upon request, although the patient has the ability to make the necessary component movements and is able to understand the request. An example is the patient who cannot put out his tongue on request but can lick his lips when it is suggested that his mouth looks dry. Patients with lesions affecting the dominant hemisphere, which cause aphasia, may have apraxia affecting the limbs. When asked to salute, brush his teeth, or comb his hair, the patient is unable to do so. The stimulus that fails to elicit a response is verbal.

*Constructional apraxia.* This is most easily tested by asking the patient to draw a simple picture such as the face of a clock or a flower. Spontaneous drawing is better than copying an already drawn figure, although both tests will give information. Patients who have a severe defect in constructional ability may have difficulty finding their way about their city or neighborhood or even their own house. These defects are seen particularly with nondominant (nearly always right) parietal lobe lesions, with or without a prominent neglect syndrome.

*Agnosia.* This defect is a failure to recognize objects, pictures, or spatial relationships, over and above any defect in the primary visual system (usual) or the somesthetic system (rare). A patient may not recognize the faces of relatives, but can identify them when they speak. He may not recognize a coin held in front of him, but readily recognizes it by touch. In patients with visual agnosia, there is often an associated defect in cortically directed eye movements and some degree of hemianopia. Note that confusional states (see the section on awareness and personality) can also produce defects in visual recognition.

## The Patient in Coma

A patient suffering from a disease producing stupor or coma requires particular types of neurological assessment, although the general principles of the examination are unaltered. Efforts should be made to define the level of consciousness, to localize the site of the lesion causing the disturbance, and to establish the levels of the brain that are functioning and those that are nonfunctioning. The clinician must develop certain skills in observation and assessment of patients in stuporous or comatose states, because the parts of the neurological examination that require patient cooperation are obviously unavailable to him. Therefore, various clues, minor observations, and impressions must be relied upon in their stead. Certain observations are of such paramount importance that they should receive special attention.*

1. The eye movements of a comatose patient should be very critically observed. In patients with bilateral hemisphere disease, in whom the brain stem and pontine structures are functioning, roving eye movements are common. The eyes will drift from side to side. When the head is passively turned, the eyes respond reflexly and move from side to side or up and down in a conjugate manner (doll's eye movements). If one labyrinth is irrigated with cold water in the ear canal, the eyes will drift conjugately toward that side. The cold water produces a convection current in the labyrinthine

*Fred Plum and Jerome B. Posner, *Diagnosis of Stupor and Coma*, 3rd ed. (Philadelphia: F. A. Davis, 1980).

canals, causing vestibular hypofunction resulting in this movement. With deterioration of function, there is a so-called rostro-caudal degeneration of neural function; the eye movements become less conjugate, and lateral or up and down movements are less easy to elicit. In patients with brain stem or pontine dysfunction, natural roving eye movements as well as reflex elicited eye movements become impaired and finally lost. On the side of a pontine lesion, lateral eye movements to that side are impossible no matter what the stimulus.

Dysconjugate eye movements—whether those of a divergence with failure of adduction, which is a common feature of a lesion of median longitudinal fasciculus, or those with a nystagmus, asymmetric eye movements, or other abnormalities—are strong indicators of midbrain or pontine disorder.

2. Pupillary functions should be carefully checked. Asymmetric pupils should be noted. They may have a number of causes, such as Horner's syndrome, third nerve dysfunction, or damage to the ciliary ganglion. In patients who have damage to the midbrain (a common occurrence in herniation of the temporal lobe) dysfunction is common, often accompanied by third nerve deficit on the side of the herniating lesion. This oculomotor damage will produce, in sequence, slight constriction of the pupil, then dilatation of the pupil on that side, followed by lateral deviation of the eye and ptosis.

Pupillary reflexes may also be markedly changed by pharmacological effects, and it must be established whether opiates, atropine, and various other medication have been used, because they may cause dilated, fixed, or small pupils. Small pupils, in the absence of a pharmacological cause, indicate bilateral Horner's syndrome such as is observed in a pontine hemorrhage interrupting the descending sympathetic fibers.

3. The respiratory pattern in the patient who is stuporous or comatose may be strongly indicative of the level of the lesion and its severity. Normal, regular respirations are observed in patients who have bilateral hemisphere dysfunction, which does not interrupt brain stem and pontine reflex control of respiration. Patients with bilateral hemisphere disease, whether structural or related to a metabolic disorder, may develop Cheyne-Stokes respiration, a regular, alternating pattern in which periods of hyperventilation are gradually followed by periods of apnea, followed by restoration and the gradual building-up of hyperventilation. Cheyne-Stokes respiration is common in patients with a number of different causes of supranuclear, that is, bilateral hemisphere, disorder. Patients with lesions of the pons typically have irregular, erratic breathing, sometimes called ataxic respirations. In late stages, gasping or very short cycle respiration may occur. Rarely, central neurogenic hyperventilation, apparently caused most frequently by lesions of the periaqueductal gray matter, may be observed. Loss of respiratory control or defective breathing may require immediate assisted ventilation.

4. Assessment of motor function of a patient in coma follows the same rules as the assessment of motor function in awake patients. Efforts should be made to establish whether or not the patient has abnormalities of tone and whether the extremities will move in response to various stimuli. In particular, it is important to note whether the movements appear to be reflex in origin or to have some psychologically interpretable cause. The patient should be observed for spontaneous movements, for restless changes in position, and for efforts to move a limb into a more comfortable position, observations that strongly suggest that the patient is restlessly stuporous rather than comatose. One-sided abnormalities of movement

should be carefully searched for. Patients with a hemiparesis who are comatose may show nothing more than a slight asymmetry of movement in response to noxious stimuli or to changes in positioning of the body. Reflexes and plantar responses should naturally be tested, but asymmetries of these reflexes are frequently difficult to discern and are often less reliable than observations of spontaneous or reflex movement.

Decerebrate rigidity and decorticate states should be particularly looked for in a comatose patient. These postures may occur spontaneously. If they do not, the patient should be stimulated, typically by rubbing the sternum with one's knuckles or by pressing the supraorbital ridge to produce noxious stimuli. Decerebrate regidity is a characteristic feature of high midbrain dysfunction, typically seen with herniation of the temporal lobe and lateral compression of the midbrain. It may also occur in some drug-induced states and in cerebral anoxia and in expanding posterior fossa lesions such a cerebellar hemorrhage.

The patient in coma may also be assessed by means of EEG, which may indicate the degree of cerebral function, but the clinical examination is more likely to be conclusive.

## Description of a Convulsive Attack

In attempting to assess the nature of a fit, whether witnessed or described by a witness or by the patient, the first point to be ascertained is whether true loss of consciousness occurred. The patient should be questioned as to whether there is a blank in his memory and whether the gap is absolute or whether some hazy memory of voices or movement remains. The person who observed the attack is questioned as to the patient's behavior in the critical period. Did he lie limp and still, or were there spasms or movements? If there were spasms or movements, were they coordinated and purposive, directed toward persons or objects, or were they bizarre and purposeless?

During an attack, a trained observer will note the nature of the movements, particularly any one-sidedness, and the direction of movement of the head and eyes, at the same time watching change in color, as he places some firm object (e.g., the handle of a spoon with several turns of cloth around it) between the patient's teeth to prevent him from biting his tongue. He will then examine the corneal reflexes and pupils. As any convulsion that is present subsides, he might examine the knee jerks and plantar responses, and note if incontinence has occurred. The mode of recovery of consciousness and co-operation, as well as the mode of onset, may provide useful information. If hysteria is suspected, the reaction to a painful stimulus, e.g., pricking with a pin, or strong pinch of the tendo achillis, may be observed during the attack.

The following list summarizes the information which one should attempt to obtain as soon as possible after the attack from the nurse or other observer:

1. What was the patient doing just before the attack (occupation, any special emotional or physical stress, any peculiar attitude or constriction of neck or prolonged lack of food)?
2. The patient's general condition before the attack—asleep, awake, irritable, dull, etc.?
3. Onset—sudden or gradual? Falling?
4. Cry or noise?
5. Did the observer consider the patient unconscious? Why? Duration of unconsciousness?

6. Color of face—pale, flushed, blue, natural, etc.?
7. Movements, if any? Any stiffness of the limbs, their position, any jerkings or twitching? Any purposive movements such as clutching at objects or observer, or fighting, kicking, avoiding examination?
8. Turning of head or eyes? If so, to which side?
9. Was the attack generalized? If not, which part was first affected and in what order did any spread occur? Which side was most affected?
10. Duration of movements?
11. Biting of the tongue?
12. Incontinence of urine or feces?
13. Symptoms after the attack (headache, sleep, vomiting, peculiar behavior, weeping, or other emotional disturbance)?

A typical epileptic convulsion shows tonic and clonic phases. The muscles first involved are thrown into a spasm that may last many seconds (tonic phase), then begin to relax periodically for longer and longer intervals, so that the spasm becomes broken up into jerks repeated once or twice a second, then more slowly (clonic phase) before ceasing. The involved part then remains limp and motionless for a time before natural movement returns. Different parts may be involved serially, so that the arm, for example, may be showing clonic jerks when the head and eyes begin to turn in tonic phase. The first part involved in tonic phase indicates the focus of the attack. In generalized attacks the body muscles may be first involved, causing an expiratory cry. Turning of the head and eyes at onset points to a frontal focus on the side opposite the direction of turning. In minor attacks, a sudden jerk or flexion of both arms may be the only sign of convulsion. In myoclonic epilepsy, irregular twitchings begin to appear in one or other part and gradually become more prominent and frequent before the tonic phase begins. Status epilepticus is defined as a series of attacks without recovery of consciousness in the intervals, but in this sense is only a severe degree of grouped epileptic attacks. Jacksonian epilepsy is a progressive march of the convulsion from a part that is first involved to related parts, each of which is convulsed in turn. Such an attack points to a closely circumscribed focus of origin. Focal epilepsy, where one side is involved before the other, has less specifically localizing significance. The aura is of high localizing value, as are sucking movements and smacking of the lips. Postictal automatic behavior, such as undressing in public, irritability, or other unusual behavior, is due to incomplete recovery of consciousness. After a series of convulsions in one limb or one side, there may be an exhaustion paralysis (Todd's postepileptic hemiplegia) after full recovery of other function.

## Special Investigations

### Lumbar Puncture

The purpose of lumbar puncture is to ascertain if the pressure or contents of the cerebrospinal fluid are changed or the subarachnoid space obstructed, sometimes to introduce diagnostic or therapeutic agents into close relationship with the nervous system, or (rarely) to relieve abnormal accumulation of fluid. Lumbar puncture is contraindicated when infection of the skin or subcutaneous tissues in the path of the needle would risk transfer of infection to the subarachnoid space. It is also contraindicated when more than slight headache or papilledema indicate considerable increase of intracranial pressure. In such cases, special precautions are necessary if it is vital to secure information as to the state of the spinal fluid. It is important to remember not to depend on papilledema as a sign of increased intracranial pressure in the elderly.

Though the measurement of pressure is unnecessary in some diagnostic and therapeutic procedures, pressure enters the differential diagnosis of so many cases of nervous disease that it is an advantage to use a manometer routinely in diagnostic puncture.

*Technique*

The needle most commonly used is made of 21-gauge steel with a stylet. After measuring the pressure in a manometer, fluid is collected after withdrawal of the stylet. The metal should be pliable enough to bend without danger of breaking. Too small a gauge obstructs flow and pressure. A shorter needle can be used with children, and in infants a blood sampling needle may be used.

Lumbar puncture is not without discomfort and even danger in some respects, and care should be taken of the specimen of fluid to see that all necessary examinations are performed, to avoid having to repeat the procedure unnecessarily. It is of the utmost importance to maintain the most complete asepsis of the needle, for the subarachnoid space can be infected, with results that may be tragic.

The patient should be reassured while being arranged in position. He should lie on one side, his knees drawn up to the abdomen, his neck flexed forward. This posture opens the intervertebral spaces, and it is useful to have the patient clasp his hands under his knees at this stage. His back should lie along the edge of the bed or table, the pelvis vertical. The lumbar spinous processes are then palpated. An imaginary line between the tips of the iliac crests crosses the spine between the third and fourth lumbar spinous processes, and this is the most favorable site for puncture. In adipose patients it is useful to mark the position of the uppermost iliac crest with a dab of iodine. The skin over the whole lumbar spine is carefully disinfected, either with soap and water followed by alcohol or with tincture of iodine. If iodine is used, it should be removed by alcohol after the puncture to avoid skin reactions. A sterile towel is draped to cover the edge of bed or table. The operator's hands are thoroughly cleansed by scrubbing with soap and water.

The operator, wearing sterile gloves, sits on a stool and again defines the third-fourth interspace. The skin at this point is infiltrated with local anesthetic through a hypodermic needle, raising a wheal. A stronger 2-inch needle is then attached to the syringe and about 5 cc. of anesthetic infiltrated into the subcutaneous tissue and underlying interspinous ligament down to the bone.

The lumbar puncture needle, with stylet inserted so as to leave no hollow at the point, is now taken up and held firmly by the hilt. It should be inserted at right angles to the skin and pushed firmly and steadily through the thickened wheal. The operator must not touch the point. Placing the left thumb firmly below the third-fourth interspace just before introducing the needle avoids displacement of the skin during puncture. When the needle has penetrated the skin, it is steadily advanced at right angles to the vertical plane but tilted very slightly away from the patient's head. It should thus enter in the midline and slightly under the third spine. After some three centimeters or more, depending on the thickness of the lumbar muscles, a slight "give" is felt as the needle pierces the ligamentum flavum.

The stylet is now withdrawn to determine if the meninges have also been punctured. If fluid does not appear, gentle advance of the needle for a further few millimeters will pierce the dura, and fluid may be obtained. If hard resistance is felt at any point, bone has been encountered and the needle should be withdrawn to the subcutaneous tissues and alignment rechecked before again inserting it. To the experienced operator the "give" of the ligament is characteristic, and if fluid is not obtained within a few millimeters of this point, the needle is rotated slightly to eliminate the possibility that a membrane lies flat against its opening. It should not be necessary to advance the needle more than two centimeters after penetrating the ligament, for the extradural venous plexus is then likely to be damaged, and blood will contaminate the puncture.

If the patient complains of pain shooting down one leg, the needle has deviated from the midline and a nerve root has been struck. Besides insufficient flexion of the spine and deviation from the midline, the commonest cause of failure to obtain fluid is blunting of the point of the needle, which should be carefully inspected. If the needle is dull, it pushes the dura forward and compresses the meningeal sac. This occurs frequently with the soft metal disposable needles in most disposable kits. It is important to avoid damage to the intervertebral disc by inserting the needle too deeply. When a drop of clear fluid indicates successful puncture, the stylet is immediately replaced to prevent further loss, and the patient is instructed to relax. He should be reassured that he will feel no further pain, and he should unclasp his hands and loosen the posture of his legs and abdomen. The manometer is then fitted to the needle, and the stopcock is turned to direct the flow into the manometer. An assistant may hold the top of the manometer to steady it. If the patient's pelvis is vertical, the manometer should also be vertical.

Any strained posture or holding of respiration by the patient will distend the venous system and artificially raise the spinal fluid pressure, and since the true resting pressure is the first observation to be made, absolute relaxation is essential. The patient's head should be supported on pillows so it is level with the needle. If the fluid is in free communication, the level of spinal fluid in the manometer should show small cardiac and respiratory pulsations. If these do not occur or if the pressure rises only very slowly, try a slight rotation of the needle, or an advance of two or three mm. When a steady level is maintained, note the pressure registered. If it is 200 mm. or higher, be certain that the patient is relaxed by inspecting his posture, watching his breathing, and by engaging him in conversation. If there is any doubt as to free communication between needle and subarachnoid space, get the patient to cough or strain, or have an assistant press on his abdomen with the palm of the hand, any of which procedures should cause a transitory rise in pressure.

If there is a question of a spinal cord lesion which may be compressive, then dynamics can be performed. In most general hospitals, with the presence of excellent neuroradiological facilities, neurosurgical consultation and myelography will be done directly. If there is a question whether these should be done or if they are not available, dynamics remains the most practical way to establish spinal cord compression. It is desirable to always have cervical and thoracic spine films beforehand to establish the level of potential lesion prior to this testing.

To demonstrate that the spinal subarachnoid space is not obstructed by compression at some level, observe the effect of compression of the jugular veins on the resting lumbar puncture pressure. The distension of the cerebral veins thus caused raises the intracranial pressure, and this rise is normally transmitted directly to the lumbar manometer. If no change occurs in the lumbar manometer, or the rise and fall in pressure is very delayed, the lumbar sac does not communicate with the cranial subarachnoid space (spinal block, Queckenstedt's test). Pressure on the abdomen and straining should still cause a rise by distension of the spinal veins below the lesion. An assistant should compress and release the jugular veins gently when requested, taking care not to cause pain by undue pressure, yet to hold the fingers close to the trachea so as to include the internal jugulars. *This test should not be performed when it is already clear that intracranial pressure is over 200 mm.* The effect of compression of each jugular separately is seldom of value except in lateral sinus thrombosis (Ayer-Toby test), owing to great variation in the venous drainage to one or other side.

The application of a sphygmomanometer cuff around the neck is a more gentle method of compression and is less likely to cause wincing or abdominal strain. When the cuff is in place, the resting pressure is noted at 10-second intervals. After 30 seconds the cuff is quickly inflated to 40 mm. mercury, and held at this pressure for 20 seconds. The pressure is then suddenly released. The lumbar pressures are noted at 10-second intervals. The findings are recorded in a graph, charting the observed pressures against 10-second intervals on the baseline, the moments of application and release of cuff pressure being shown by arrows. A delay in fall of pressure (ball-valve block) is often important in establishing the presence of partial spinal block.

Since the spinal canal in the cervical region is greatly altered by movements of the neck, these spinal dynamics should be recorded, first with the neck flexed and then with the neck extended, when there is any question of cervical cord compression. It is important to avoid obstruction of the jugular veins by the posturing, for this would vitiate the test.

Whether or not dynamics has been done, one should always check what happens as fluid is withdrawn. When the pressure relationships of the cerebrospinal fluid have been noted, fluid may be allowed to flow slowly from the needle and the pressure recorded after the collection of each 2 cc. Sudden cessation of flow is probably due to occlusion of the needle by a root or membrane, and partial rotation of the needle should free it. A rapid fall of pressure after removal of a small amount of fluid indicates a small reservoir, such as occurs in expanding cerebral lesions or in herniation at the foramen magnum or tentorial opening. If along with this rapid fall there is any other indication of increased intracranial pressure, the puncture should be terminated and the patient returned to bed with head low and feet raised. A slow fall of pressure during the removal of large amounts of fluid indicates an excess of spinal fluid, as in external hydrocephalus, meningitis, or meningism.

In most cases, 4-5 cc. of fluid are sufficient for all tests. If there is any suspicion of increased intracranial pressure, no further fluid should be removed when the pressure has dropped to 100 mm. If the fluid is bloodstained, it is advisable to collect a last specimen in a separate tube. A diminished blood content in this specimen indicates that the needle has damaged a vessel. After a final pressure reading, the needle is removed, the skin puncture swabbed with alcohol or iodine, pressed gently for a few moments to control any oozing, then covered by a Band-Aid.

The patient should be kept flat in bed for 8 hours to lessen leakage through the dural puncture. If lumbar puncture headache develops, it will be worse on sitting up or standing and may be assumed to be due to leakage through the tear in the dura. The foot of the bed should be raised and fluid intake increased for 24-48 hours.

## Pathological Changes

*Pressure.* Any pressure over 200 mm. requires explanation. Low pressures may result from dehydration, leakage of fluid, or encystment of the lumbar sac. Raised pressures may be due to (1) any physiological or pathological increase of venous pressure with resulting obstruction of absorption; (2) a rapidly expanding space-occupying lesion in the cerebrum (hemorrhage, edema, tumor, abscess); (3) a slowly growing intracranial mass obstructing the circulation of the fluid by anatomical distortion or compression; or (4) excessive formation of fluid, such as occurs in meningitis or meningism.

*Appearance of the fluid.* Normally the fluid is clear and colorless. It may be bloody in cases of cerebral trauma, cerebral hemorrhage, subarachnoid hemorrhage, and "bloody tap" (puncture of vertebral or thecal veins by the needle). The supernatant fluid is xanthochromic (yellowish) in all fluids in which the blood has been present more than three or four hours before the puncture. Xanthochromia is shown if there has recently been a leakage of blood into the subarachnoid spaces, in cases of severe jaundice, and in all fluids with a high protein content, as occurs commonly in subarachnoid block, acute and chronic meningitis, and occasionally in brain tumor. The fluid is turbid, cloudy, "ground glass," or purulent in appearance when many cells are present. Degenerated polymorphonuclear leukocytes are more apt to give a purulent appearance to the fluid than fresh leukocytes or lymphocytes. A coarse clot forms in the fluid from cases of acute meningitis. A fine cobweb clot occurs in practically all cases of tuberculous meningitis and in many cases of syphilitic meningitis, yeast meningitis, and more rarely in poliomyelitis, syphilis of the nervous system, brain tumor, and other conditions. There is rarely sufficient fibrin present to cause the fluid to clot into a jelly.

*Cells.* One drop of a ½ percent solution of methylene blue is added to 1 cc. of the fluid and shaken. A drop of the mixture is placed in the counting chamber. If the cells are few, several mm³ should be counted. Particular care should be taken to distinguish between red cells, lymphocytes, and polymorphonuclears.

The normal cell count is 0 to 5 cells per cubic millimeter, all lymphocytes. An increase in the cell count results from any process causing an inflammatory reaction of the meninges or ependyma. Such an inflammatory reaction is most commonly caused by a bacterial, viral, or syphilitic infection of the central nervous system. It may also occur as a result of an inflammatory reaction of the meninges overlying a focus of infection in the cranial cavity, such as mastoid disease or other osteitis, extradural or cerebral abscess, or a necrotic focus resulting from brain tumors, cerebral hemorrhage, or softenings, especially when such changes approach the lining of the ventricle. The cells in the fluid are usually of hematogenous origin, but occasionally cells derived from the perivascular spaces or the arachnoid may be found. Polymorphonuclear leukocytes usually are the predominating cell type in acute meningeal inflammations; lymphocytes and plasma cells in chronic inflammations. Rarely, tumor cells or other abnormal cells may be found in the fluid in cases with tumors of the brain or leukemic infiltrations. Specific cell types, including tumor cells, can be easily identified with the cytocentrifuge techniques usually available in hospital laboratories.

*Protein.* The normal protein content of the fluid varies between 15 and 45 mg. per 100 ml. An increase in the protein content occurs by transudation of protein through the vessels of the meninges or the choroid plexus as a result of their increased permeability. Such an increase is most commonly found in cases with an acute or chronic meningitis and is also frequently seen in cases with tumors near the ventricles or with vascular growths and occasionally in cases with degenerative lesions of the central nervous system. The most marked increase in protein content occurs in cases with subarachnoid block when the loculation syndrome of Froin is present. In such cases the fluid is yellow, spontaneously clotting, and may have a protein content as high as 3,500 to 5,000 mg. per 100 ml.

*Sugar.* The normal glucose content of the cerebrospinal fluid varies between 50 and 80 mg. per 100 ml. An increase in the sugar content is not significant of any abnormality of the central nervous system but is merely indicative of an increased serum sugar content. A decrease in the sugar content of the cerebrospinal fluid usually accompanies infection of the meninges. Other meningeal processes, such as sarcoidosis, also can lower it. A decrease in sugar content may occasionally occur as the result of hypoglycemia and rarely is seen in cases with bloody or purulent cerebrospinal fluids which do not contain bacteria.

*Gamma globulin.* The gamma globulin may be elevated in certain disorders such as multiple sclerosis and other demyelinating diseases. This can be measured chemically or by electrophoresis. Myelin basic protein is a myelin fraction seen after acute damage to myelin and correlates with active demyelination or destruction.

## CT Scan

*Definition.* A CT (computerized tomography) scan is a laminographic technique using X-ray as the source of radiation. The absorption indices of these layers are then computed. The machinery currently in use gives definition of sections of the cranium approximately 13 mm. in thickness, so that under ordinary circumstances six or seven different sections are demonstrated. The technique is excellent for detecting differences in density caused by tumor, hemorrhage, atrophy, or infarction.

*Indications.* CT scanning is indicated for the detection of tumors or hemorrhage either in the brain or in the extracerebral spaces. It may be used acutely, and the availability of the technique in hospitals has markedly changed the management of patients with hemorrhage or tumor because of its precision, speed, and lack of serious complications. The technique may also be used as an outpatient investigation and for long-term follow-up of patients with chronic atrophic lesions, hydrocephalus, or seizure disorders.

*Contraindications.* CT scanning is ordinarily accompanied by the infusion of a radiopaque substance, such as that used for intravenous pyelography, and some patients are allergic to the iodine-containing compound, so that anaphylaxis may rarely occur. CT scanning, like any diagnostic procedure, may produce misleading results, and there are situations in which undue reliance upon the technique has led to serious errors in diagnosis.

Electroencephalography

*Definition.* This technique gives a paper record of the electrical potentials generated from the brain which can be recorded over the skull. It is particularly useful for demonstrating epileptic discharges, especially during the interictal period when the epileptic tendency may be very obvious on EEG and confirm this clinical diagnosis. Earlier uses of the EEG, related to localization of brain tumors or infarctions and to demonstration of minor abnormalities in patients with psychiatric disorder, have begun to be superseded by other forms of testing.

*Indications.* EEG testing is indicated for patients with convulsive disorder or forms of paroxysmal activity of the brain. It is a useful screening test for patients with headache or dizziness. On some occasions it is useful for detection of the level of consciousness in patients with a metabolic encephalopathy or other generalized disorders of the brain. It can be useful to define the adequacy of dialysis in renal patients or the effectiveness of treatment of other metabolic disorders. In some hospitals the EEG is used to detect electrocerebral silence, thereby defining "brain death," but this use has not become obligatory, and changes in this usage are to be expected.

*Contraindications.* None.

*Risks and dangers.* None.

## Opaque Myelography

*Definition.* Opaque myelography is the demonstration of the spinal subarachnoid space and structures outlined in it. A small volume of cerebrospinal fluid is replaced with a radio-opaque solution, either an oily insoluble compound such as Pantopaque or water-soluble compound such as Amipaque.

*Indications.* The most common use for opaque myelography is to demonstrate a potentially compressive lesion of the cord or spinal roots. This may be a tumor, a prolapsed disc, cervical spondylosis, or any of a number of other lesions. The myelography may be merely lumbar, when it is known that the lesion is in the lumbar roots, or the dye may be carried up to the cervical region for a full demonstration of the entire subarachnoid space.

*Contraindications.* 1. Known inflammatory reaction or subarachnoid hemorrhage around the cord or of the meninges. 2. A lesion of the cerebral hemispheres or in the posterior fossa, which potentially could cause herniation by means of change in pressure with the lumbar puncture.

*Complications and risks.* 1. Herniation of the brain, as noted above. 2. Some patients with complete spinal block may become worse following lumbar puncture. If a complete block is suspected, a neurosurgical consultation should first be obtained, or if this is unexpectedly found at myelography, neurosurgical opinion should be obtained immediately. 3. If Pantopaque is not removed, it is a potential source of irritation and may in rare cases be a cause of inflammatory arachnoiditis. 4. The Amipaque currently in use potentially may cause seizures in rare patients, particularly when the dye enters the cranial cavity. Other patients have complications of severe nausea, headache, and vomiting following the use of water-soluble contrast media. Usually these symptoms are brief, lasting no more than 12-24 hours. 5. Any patient who has a myelogram or any other form of lumbar puncture may be subject to spinal headaches, which may last for several weeks and are worsened by being erect.

## Angiography

*Definition.* Cerebral angiography is a technique of opacification of blood vessels. The standard methods in use involve catheterization of these vessels, usually from a femoral artery, or less commonly from the right brachial artery. The common carotid, internal carotid, external carotid, or vertebral arteries may be catheterized and selectively injected with contrast medium.

*Indications.* Angiography is particularly indicated for detection and definition of cerebral arteriovenous malformations, berry aneurysms, and brain tumors. Selective angiography may be highly useful in localizing and defining the blood supply of these lesions. In addition, angiography of the carotid circulation in the neck may be useful in defining internal carotid stenosis or occlusion as related to transient ischemic attacks or cerebral infarction in the carotid territory. Under rare circumstances, vertebral angiography may be required to define the angiographic anatomy related to vertebral basilar ischemic attacks.

*Contraindications.* Patients with fever, coma, increased intracranial pressure, and patients who are restless or combative do poorly in angiography and are much more likely to have complications. These states, therefore, are relative contraindications to angiographic investigation.

*Dangers.* There are several dangers in angiography, constituting an overall risk of approximately 1 percent. These include development of a cerebral infarction related to embolization, thrombosis of some portion of the arterial supply, sensitivity to the angiographic contrast media, and various forms of cortical blindness or encephalopathy, presumably related to overall change in blood circulation. Many of these complications are temporary, but there is an established, small but apparently irreducible risk of serious infarction or death.

## Electromyography and Nerve Conduction

*Definition.* Electromyography (EMG) consists of recording the electrical potentials of muscle fibers by means of a needle placed within the muscle. At rest, normal skeletal muscle shows no electrical activity. In various types of damage to muscle fibers, such as myopathies, dystrophies, and myositis, small potentials indicate a loss of muscle fibers from each motor unit. In diseases of nerve, such as nerve root disease, amyotrophic lateral sclerosis, and polyneuropathy, the pattern of potentials on electromyography may show small fibrillation potentials, indicating neural atrophy; reinnervation potentials, which are large and polyphasic; or fasciculations, indicating discharge of large or normal motor units.

Nerve conduction testing consists of recording the muscle action potentials over muscles following nerve stimulation, or recording the nerve potentials themselves. Following stimulation, by means of recording from several different sites along the course of the nerve, the conduction velocity of the fast conducting fibers in that nerve can be computed. In addition, the total number of responsive axons can be computed by measuring the height of the action potential.

*Indications.* EMG and nerve conduction are useful tests when there is disease of the peripheral nervous system. This may consist of root disorders, such as cervical or lumbar herniated disc, or polyneuropathy or primary disease of muscle. In some circumstances, the demonstration of a normal EMG and nerve conduction may help to decide that a patient's symptoms represent psychogenic disease.

*Contraindications.* The EMG needles are painful, and the nerve stimulation as part of nerve conduction is also unpleasant. The patient should be warned of this aspect, and in some circumstances patients are unable to tolerate the tests.

*Risks and dangers.* No permanent or lasting sequelae are known.

## Evoked Potentials

*Definition.* These are also tests of nerve conduction. A form of visual, auditory, or somatosensory stimulation is applied, and the speed of conduction is measured through the nervous system. The tests require specialized equipment and oscilloscopes capable of averaging potentials and computing small potentials which are difficult to record.

*Indications.* These tests are useful primarily for detecting demyelination in the nervous system. Demyelination causes a characteristic form of slowing of these potentials, which would support the diagnosis of multiple sclerosis or some other form of demyelinating disease. In some circumstances the reduction in a potential or absence of a potential without slowing is useful, and this has been used to follow the course of spinal cord injury. This specialized use is not widespread.

*Contraindications, risks, and dangers.* None.

## Roentgenograms of Skull and Spine

In the skull, learn to recognize normal and abnormal variations of the sella turcica, thinning of the vault due to chronic disease or pressure, erosion and localized deposition of bone due to disease or tumor, and the appearances of trauma. The pituitary fossa and its clinoid processes are best seen in stereoscopic or tomographic views, which are also essential for detailed study of skull markings and texture. Learn to recognize the difference between a large but normal sella turcica and one which is "opened out" by internal pressure. The vascular markings of the skull deserve special study, for they are subject to great variation in normal health, yet a localized increase may be the only clue to meningeal tumor or vascular malformation. In the spine note the wedging of a collapsed vertebra, the erosion of disease (the clean, punched-out erosion of neoplasm, and the irregular calcification commonly seen at the margins of erosion by inflammatory disease), the widened vertebral canal or intervertebral foramen due to benign, slow-growing tumors. Learn to recognize the pedicles and the posterior intervertebral joints. Note the obscuration of outline of the latter in true spondylitis and the lack of significance of calcification in the anterior spinal ligament (spurs —compare calcified costal cartilage). Use tomography liberally to help define areas not well seen on routine X-rays because of overlapping shadows.

## Biopsy

Biopsy may yield important information in the following circumstances in neurological cases:

1. Identification of a muscular atrophy as being either a primary dystrophy, a myositis, or simple neural degeneration.
2. Identification of nodular inflammation due to periarteritis nodosa, gummatous syphilis, thromboangitis, or temporal arteritis.
3. Identification of muscular or subcutaneous parasites (cysticercosis, trichina).
4. Identification of type of thickening of peripheral cutaneous nerves (neurofibromatosis, chronic hypertrophic interstitial neuritis, amyloid disease).

Biopsy for identification of muscular atrophy should be in a carefully chosen recently wasted muscle. In severe wasting, nothing but remnants may be seen. On the other hand, few muscles may be affected, and it is important to choose one that is affected. The muscle fibers excised should not be stretched, and immediately after excision should be gently spread on a piece of stiff paper or card and allowed to adhere to it, and the piece of paper with attached muscle fixed in formol saline or Zenker's fixative. The paper will prevent the muscle from contracting into a knotted lump and thus will allow good histological sections.

Biopsy for any nodular disease included under points 2 and 3 above should aim to secure a nodule. Otherwise it is a waste of time and effort.

Biopsy for cutaneous nerves should be made only on some relatively unimportant nerve, such as lesser internal cutaneous, sural, external cutaneous of the thigh, or dorsal nerve of the foot, and the nerve should be palpably enlarged. The excised piece should also be laid straight on a piece of card and allowed to adhere before fixation in formol saline.

## Tests for Autonomic Nervous Function

Lack of the sympathetic nervous supply to the skin may be seen in a rise of skin temperature, lack of pilomotor response to skin stimulation or pinch of trapezius muscle, and absence of sweating in the area concerned. To demonstrate the change in skin temperature, the patient must be cooled, for when the surroundings are at or above body temperature the affected skin may be cooler than the rest. The pilomotor response is irregular and often difficult to provoke.

One can plot out the area of sweat abnormality on sensory charts. Areas of decreased sweating can be measured by a finger moving over the dry skin, electrical measurements of skin resistance, or by special testing such as starch and iodine applied to surface areas.